Book cover by Onur Burconur

Book design by Alex Holguin

Illustrations by Jamie Mills & Alex Holguin

Images used under license from Shutterstock.com

Vol. 1 edition 2023

To all of my fellow pre- and post-op bariatric babes—
*In case no one in your life has said these words to you before, let me be the first to say I'm really f*cking proud of you for choosing weight loss surgery. Not because you chose to lose weight, but because you chose to change your life, and I think that's really beautiful and brave.*

To all my fellow bariatric practitioners and colleagues—
Thank you for all you do for me, our community, and your patients. Your patients and clients are so lucky to have you, and I'm very grateful you are here to listen and continue to learn.

To partners, family members, and friends of beloved bariatric babes—
Thank you for being there for the person you love on this journey. While they might feel alone at times, the fact that you are there to support them reaffirms that they are. in fact, not alone. And while they are going through immense change, so are you, and I'm proud of you for allowing them the space they need to navigate this chapter as you navigate it too. I hope this book helps you to better understand and support your person through their journey, as well as give yourself a better understanding of the process.

And to anyone who is skeptical and maybe even critical of bariatrics—
I applaud you for being here. Thank you for being open to understanding and hearing another viewpoint. Thank you for choosing to read my words, hear patients' voices, and take the action steps to bring us one step closer to closing the gap on our opposing viewpoints.

Table Of Contents

Foreword

by Dr. Eric Smith, DO FASMBS, Medical Director of Kentucky Bariatric Institute, Medical Director of Robotics and Bariatrics for Lifepoint Health, and Bariatric surgeon featured on TLC's 1000-Lb. Sisters

I remember as far back as my surgical residency hearing my trainers say, "If you are really paying attention, you will learn as much from your patients as you do from us." There were times I understood what they meant, but I also wondered if it was just one of the hundreds of cliché statements they threw our way in the midst of the grind of surgical residency while we worked 100 plus hours a week. As I started my practice, I began to see what they meant.

I saw how treatments affected patients. I began to not only see the outcome, but also to learn more important lessons. I saw the impact of patience and empathy and realized that surgical decision-making was important, but how it was applied, delivered, and communicated often determined the ultimate outcome.

I started in practice as a general and bariatric surgeon in 2006, and over the years, the role of social media in medicine has evolved significantly. I watched this evolution and was adamant I wanted no part of it. For much of my early career, I saw it as a threat to healthy information. How could this be better than what I was telling my patients? I am the physician; patients shouldn't be getting advice or opinion from sources that were not fact-checked or backed by legitimate data—or were they?

I continued my resistance to what I thought was nothing but the threat of Dr. Google, until I had a good friend who understood the space sit me down and ask if I was aware of the community for bariatric surgery that was out there. I began to search through social media and was amazed at the number of accounts that not only featured surgeons, therapists, and dietitians, but also so many patients sharing their journeys of weight loss surgery too. They were sharing the highs and the lows, the non-scale victories, the struggles with body dysmorphia, the victories in finding health, and all the lessons along the way.

One of the accounts I discovered early on was @thesleeveddietitian. I was intrigued and began to scan her account: Jamie Mills, the dietitian who had weight loss surgery. That's the first thing I saw, so I began to see what her account was all about. I saw messages of education and support. I saw a patient's perspective on some of the silly rules that had been thrown at them by surgeons over the years, some of which had no scientific basis behind it and were things we did because that's what we were told to do. I enjoyed the perspective, and I was reassured by how often her followers were instructed to check with their surgeon about some of the questions that they had.

For years, I had stressed to my patients how important community was in regards to compliance, accountability, and support. I encouraged my patients to attend support groups that we offered and became frustrated when many of those groups had what I felt was subpar attendance. Then I started to see Jamie's program offered 45+ support groups a month. These covered every topic I could imagine a bariatric surgery patient could ever want to know, and then I had that light-bulb moment. Of course they cover every topic patients would want to know, as they are built for patients by a patient. Didn't I remember what I learned in residency? If you can learn these valuable lessons from your patients, why would you be so blind to seeing that your own patients can learn something from patients as well?

This started a friendship that opened my eyes to the numerous resources out there for my patients. I was so impressed by the knowledge that was being shared, and I had confidence to begin to encourage my patients to seek out these resources and, specifically, Jamie Mills.

When Jamie approached me with the opportunity to write a foreword for her book, I was honored and excited to share how meeting Jamie played a role in how I viewed patient care and community. Jamie's story is one of incredible resilience, empowerment, and a relentless pursuit of health. As a dietitian who has personally undergone weight loss surgery, she brings a unique perspective that bridges the gap between personal experience and professional expertise.

In our society, discussions around weight, body image, and health often come laden with judgment and misconceptions. Jamie has faced these challenges head-on, courageously defying the stereotypes and societal pressures that come with being an obese female pursuing a career in the field of nutrition. Her journey is not just about losing weight; it is a testament to the human spirit, the strength to rise above adversity, and the unwavering belief in oneself.

Jamie possesses an unwavering commitment to promoting healthy lifestyle changes while recognizing that nutrition is not a one-size-fits-all solution. In a world filled with fad diets and quick-fix solutions, Jamie emphasizes the importance of tailoring dietary choices to individual needs. Through her social media presence and her membership program, T.R.I.B.E®. (The Real Insights of Bariatric Eating), she has become a beacon of hope for countless individuals seeking guidance on their own transformative journeys.

Jamie's decision to undergo bariatric surgery was not an easy one. She opens her heart and bares her soul in this book, recounting the moments of doubt, fear, and vulnerability that accompanied her choice. She candidly shares the ups and downs she experienced during the entire process, providing invaluable insights to those who may be contemplating a similar path. Her honesty and authenticity make this book a powerful source of inspiration for anyone facing their own battles with obesity or considering bariatric surgery.

But this book is about more than just Jamie's personal journey; it is a call to action, a clarion call to raise awareness about bariatric surgery and the unique challenges faced by individuals who undergo this life-changing surgery. Through her words, she shines a light on the prejudices and stereotypes that society often attaches to those who seek surgical intervention for weight loss. She challenges us to reassess our preconceived notions and encourages compassion and understanding for those who have chosen this path to reclaim their health and well-being.

Jamie is not just a dietitian or an advocate for bariatric surgery; she is a mentor and a friend to those who have walked similar paths. Her story is a testament to the power of vulnerability, resilience, and the unwavering pursuit of one's dreams, and this book is just another example of all those things. I have no doubt that her words will resonate deeply with you, offering solace, inspiration, and practical advice to all who seek it.

As you embark on this transformative journey through the pages of Jamie's book, open your heart and mind to the immense power of self-discovery and growth. I also encourage you to share it with someone who might see bariatric surgery as a shortcut or easy way out. This book will not only help you on your weight loss journey, it may help you educate those around you as they read Jamie's story. There is nothing that would make Jamie happier than playing a small role in helping others see that surgery isn't cheating obesity, it is simply treating it! I am honored to call Jamie a peer, educator, and a friend. I could not be prouder to have a small contribution to this labor of love of Jamie's that has been a long time coming.

Embrace the challenges and triumphs that lie ahead, knowing that you are not alone. Jamie Mills is here to guide you, support you, and remind you that true transformation begins within.

Eric Smith, DO FASMBS
Medical Director of Kentucky Bariatric Institute
Medical Director of Robotics and Bariatrics for Lifepoint Health
Bariatric surgeon featured on TLC's *1000-Lb. Sisters*

Who This Book Is For

One of the comments I often get from both my fellow bariatric babes, as well as from my fellow bariatric colleagues when they read my content and blog posts is, "Wow, Jamie, I feel like you're in my head!" And I expect this book to be no different.

The beauty of my being both a bariatric patient and a bariatric professional is that I am truly able to see things from multiple angles and points of view. And I've come upon crossroads and hardships both personally and professionally on this journey too.

Because of this, this book was written with two primary audiences in mind:

1. Bariatric patients: I consider anyone who has had surgery, who is awaiting their surgery date, who is/has struggled with obesity, or who may be interested in or considering bariatrics to be a "bariatric patient" for the purposes of this book. Throughout much of the book, as I'm addressing "you," I am speaking to you, the person on the receiving end of weight struggles.

2. Bariatric professionals: In many chapters throughout the book, I do shift gears and address my non-bariatric-patient audience. I consider bariatric surgeons, physicians, nurses/nurse practitioners, physician assistants, registered dietitians, clinical coordinators, therapists, exercise physiologists, etc. to fall under that umbrella 0f bariatric professionals. I often speak to "you" too in this book, as the clinician or professional who supports people on this journey.

And if you are reading this and you do not fall into either of my primary audience categories, I want to say hello and welcome. I hope this book inspires you, teaches you, and gives you much to think about.

Abbreviations & Terms

Trying to sift through resources in the weight loss surgery world can feel like reading a foreign language. And if you are a part of the bariatric community online, there are lots of specific abbreviations and terms used as part of our everyday language. Some of these terms I will also use throughout this book. I will remind you of the meanings of these abbreviations as I come upon them, but I also wanted to add a list here for reference.

Abbreviations & Terms

- AGB: adjustable gastric band (i.e., lap band)
- AMA: American Medical Association
- AOMs: anti-obesity medications
- ASMBS: American Society for Metabolic and Bariatric Surgery
- BED: binge eating disorder
- BMR: basal metabolic rate
- BP: blood pressure
- CW: current weight
- DM2: type 2 diabetes mellitus
- DS: biliopancreatic diversion with duodenal switch (sometimes also referred to as "BPD")
- GI: gastrointestinal
- GIP: gastric inhibitory peptide
- GIP: glucose-dependent insulinotropic polypeptide[1]
- GLP-1: glucagon-like peptide 1 (an incretin hormone found in the body)
- GLP-1s: a class of anti-obesity medication that mimics the GLP-1 hormone
- HW: highest weight

[1] GIP is also the acronym used for both "gastric inhibitory peptide" and "glucose=dependent insulinic polypeptide," so when you see this acronym come up in other places, it's worth double=checking which GIP they're talking about. For clarity, whenever I've used this acronym in the book, I've always included the definition.)

- LW: lowest weight
- MBS: metabolic & bariatric surgery (WLS & MBS are the same thing, and these terms may be used interchangeably.)
- NSV: non-scale victory (a win that is not related to the number on the scale)
- OAGB: one anastomosis gastric bypass
- Onederland: getting under 200 lbs. on the scale
- PCOS: polycystic ovarian syndrome (an endocrine disorder affecting 5–10% of women, with obesity being a common side effect and/or symptom)
- PCP: primary care physician
- Plastics: plastic surgery
- Proffee: protein coffee (a drink enjoyed by bariatric patients and made by pouring a protein shake into their coffee)
- RD: registered dietitian
- RNY/RYGB: Roux-en-Y gastric bypass
- SADI-S: single anastomosis duodenal switch with sleeve gastrectomy
- SW: starting weight or surgery weight
- VSG: vertical sleeve gastrectomy
- WLS: weight loss surgery

The Term "Diet"

The term "diet" is used in two ways throughout this book. First, I use it to discuss the practice of restricting food for the explicit goal of weight loss, often done unhealthily. Second, I use it to mean a food regimen to follow, often medically mandated.

When using the term "diet" in the first sense, I often will notate that I am referring to a "fad diet" or a "toxic diet" mentality. This is the type of "diet" that I don't condone or suggest one follows after weight loss surgery.

When referring to the second way in which the term "diet" is used, I often will notate that I am referring to a medically prescribed post-op diet or diet regimen that is in accordance with the American Society for Metabolic and Bariatric Surgery (ASMBS) guidelines and recommendations for WLS patients' overall health, safety, and success. This is the type of "diet" that I do support and encourage people to follow after weight loss surgery.

Please keep in mind that following your prescribed post-op diet is NOT the same as following a "fad" or "crash" diet. Understanding the distinction between the two is important, especially in the context of this book.

Journal Prompts & Additional Resources

One of my main goals for writing this book and sharing it with the world is to facilitate a conversation, as well as to provide better resources to the bariatric community. Before we can have honest conversations with each other, we must have honest conversations with ourselves, which is why I encourage you to download the free materials that go along with each chapter. I have created prompts and additional resources to help guide you through this book to better support you on your journey.

There are no right or wrong answers to the questions I leave you with. I want you to allow yourself to be completely honest with yourself and your thoughts. Rather than judging or overanalyzing your answers, I want you to approach each question and each answer with curiosity.

Journaling has been an immensely helpful tool for me on my own journey, as both a patient and professional, to truly get to know myself better. A huge piece of this journey that is often overlooked is getting to know who you are at your core, as well as who you desire to be. I hope these journal prompts allow you space and new opportunities to get to know YOU. I hope these prompts and worksheets help you think about things in a new light, or perhaps allow you to revisit old thoughts in a new way. Whatever comes up, I hope these prompts serve you in some way on your journey.

Head to

www.thesleeveddietitian.com/easy or scan the QR code below to download all additional resources, materials, handouts, worksheets, and journal prompts.

QR code that can be scanned with a phone or other camera-enabled device. To access the same materials, visit www.thesleevedditition.com/easy.

Hi, I'm Jamie.

I'm the dietitian who had weight loss surgery.

It kind of sounds like an oxymoron, doesn't it? When people picture a bariatric patient, usually an image of a 500+ pound person on a reality TV show comes to mind. But if I ask you to conjure an image of a registered dietitian, most of us think of a very thin, White female eating kale. Somehow I don't think most people would assume these two images could be the same person.

I struggled with my weight my entire life. I was over 200 pounds by the time I was nine, and nearly 300 pounds by high school (and at barely 5'4", that's a lot). It never made a lot of sense why I was so overweight, even though my sister, who grew up in the same environment with the same genetics, was not. I ate healthy foods, played outside, and did normal kid things. Yet, somehow, I was still always bigger than all my peers.

I started dieting in the fifth grade and took one dangerous approach after another to lose weight. From Weight Watchers to keto (or "Atkins," as we called it in the 90s) to extreme calorie deficits, and everything in between, nothing worked. When I was 14, I was diagnosed with polycystic ovarian syndrome (PCOS), which is an endocrine disorder that leads to excessive weight gain and inability to lose weight. It explained a lot, which was validating. For the first time, I felt like it wasn't my fault that I was so overweight. But as great as it was to learn there was a reason for my weight, it didn't enable me to make the changes I needed to. Instead, it made me feel utterly worthless and completely out of control. It made me feel like I had no control over what my body did. Why bother trying to lose weight if it doesn't matter one way or the other?

I held on to that mentality until I was in college, studying English and secondary education, with a minor in art. It wasn't until I was so big I couldn't walk across campus fast enough to get to class on time that I realized something had to give. I finally decided, even if I never actually lost a pound, I needed to try. At the very least, I needed to stop gaining at such a rapid rate.

I'll bet you're waiting for me to tell you that this is the part where I realized I was going to have weight loss surgery, lose all the weight, and live happily ever after, huh? Well, I love a good Disney fairytale more than anyone (I'm a self-proclaimed Disney adult over here, after all), but sadly, no. I was still determined to "do it on my own," because having weight loss surgery was "cheating" and would signal to the world that I had given up. And I'm no quitter.

So instead, I went back to dieting. Which worked out well at first. In those beginning months, my only focus was being consistent with healthy foods and going to the gym. After a lot of consistency and hard work, I lost 50 pounds "all on my own," I would brag. Ya know, without the help of weight loss surgery, because surely doing it "naturally" is so much better.

And it was great. Until it wasn't. Remember how I mentioned how uncomfortable it felt to be out of control with my body? Well, that control I craved only grew as I lost more weight. What started off as relatively healthy, quickly turned to overly restrictive and destructive.

I began starving myself in extreme ways. I was working two jobs, going to school, and going to the gym for hours per day with nothing more than a cup of coffee and half an apple in my system. After months of not eating, my body and mind started to do some weird things. I wasn't able to sleep, and well, lack of sleep will make you go a little bonkers.

I finally ended up getting help and going to therapy. As I slowly got better and started to eat again, I realized I never wanted anyone to struggle with their weight in the ways I had. I also never wanted someone to struggle with restriction in the ways I had. I decided at that moment that I wanted to become a registered dietitian to help other people like me, who struggled with their weight. I wanted them to know that there were better ways and they were not alone.

So I changed majors, switched universities, and started over to go to school for nutrition and dietetics. It was one of the most challenging experiences I had, but I knew I could do it. For the first time, I felt like I really believed in myself. As I learned more and more about nutrition and what was actually healthy, I continued to get better and heal my own relationship with food. However, with that healing came weight gain. And by the time I had graduated with my BS in nutrition and dietetics, I was back to my highest weight.

During my dietetic internship year in 2017, I experienced so much discrimination as the "fat intern." It was brutal doing my clinical rounds in a major teaching hospital, doing the work as a dietitian, weighing nearly 300 pounds again. The looks I got were enough to make me feel like absolutely nothing, despite how hard I had worked to get there.

In December 2017, I had my weight loss surgery. I finally decided that I needed another tool. I had tried everything. I was becoming a registered dietitian for God's sake! It wasn't a lack of willpower or a lack of trying, and it certainly was not a knowledge deficit. I needed another tool, and ultimately, I deserved a better life than I was giving myself.

As I went through the grueling six-month pre-op process to have weight loss surgery, I very quickly realized how wrong I was about surgery being "easy." Even after all I had been through, this process was the hardest experience of my life.

In total I had 27 preoperative appointments. In order to get approved for surgery, I had to meet with the bariatric coordinator, scheduler, dietitian, psychologist, my PCP (primary care physician), cardiology, and pulmonology and participate in countless blood draws. Not to mention how stressful it was to have all these people monitor your weight the entire time. To top it off, there was the constant fear that someone in my life was going to "find out" what I was doing. God forbid my dietetic peers found out, as I would be ruined. What would people think of me? I couldn't handle the shame. To sum it up, not only was I stressed and overwhelmed by this incredible life change that was about to come, but I was utterly and entirely alone. Completely isolated. I often wonder how my experience might have been different had I had the support and community at the time I so badly craved.

As I was going through these pre-op appointments, I also remember thinking, "Wow, I have an education and a background in nutrition, and understanding this post-op diet is so overwhelming!" There were so many "bariatric rules" that had to be followed. It wasn't like a normal diet. Instead, it was specific. And not to mention the crazy amount of vitamins and supplements I needed to take each day. I had my surgery on December 19, 2017. It was the scariest and best thing I ever did for myself. It was overwhelming, but I had finally done it. It was during this time I turned to social media for support and inspiration. I had been fortunate enough to connect with other bariatric patients by this time, and I was starting to feel less alone and more content with my decision.

In July 2018, I finally became a registered dietitian and was down nearly 90 pounds (and would go on to lose 20+ more). Once I became an RD (registered dietitian), I announced it on Instagram, because up until this time, I didn't share with my bariatric friends what my career was.

The outpouring of support and excitement I received from the bariatric community was beyond my wildest dreams. I was worried people would judge me for being an RD who needed surgery, but instead, they were so excited I was among them. So many DMs read, "OMG, Jamie, you're a dietitian too?! Can you help me?" or "Wow, I'm so happy! Someone who actually gets it! I trust you so much, I would love your help."

It occurred to me at that moment that I was in a very unique position to use both my personal experiences AND my professional expertise to help other people. The thought of saving someone from the hardships I had experienced on my journey was enough to propel me to take the action steps needed to help others who were struggling and alone.

In 2019, I filed my LLC and officially started my nutrition coaching business, The Sleeved Dietitian®. I started off coaching individual nutrition clients, and to my pleasant surprise, I was fully booked very quickly. It occurred to me that I was in high demand and more people needed and WANTED my support and help. In 2020, I launched my bariatric membership program and since then have supported thousands of women on their bariatric journeys. It's my goal to continue to educate and inspire those in the bariatric community. I want to always be their most trusted resource and the one they go to when they feel alone. It's also my goal to continue to advocate for bariatric surgery and normalize it so more people can get the care and support they need and so badly deserve.

Introduction

Weight loss surgery is considered the gold standard for treating obesity and achieving long-term weight loss results. Nearly 42% of adults in the United States suffer from obesity.[2] Obesity is linked to over 40 other diseases and premature death.[3] Despite knowing that obesity is a complex and multifaceted disease, it is still largely viewed by society as a moral failing or a "willpower" issue.

Bariatric and metabolic surgery is the most effective treatment for obesity and can reduce risk of premature death by up to 50%. Patients who undergo bariatric surgery are anticipated to lose as much as 60–77% of their excess weight in the first two years and, on average, maintain 50% of that loss after five years. However, despite it being the most effective and best known treatment we have available, it is a procedure that is severely underutilized, with less than 1% of the current eligible surgical population taking advantage of this treatment.[4]

Why is that? How is it that the most effective treatment we have available for obesity is simultaneously the most underutilized? My guess is that if we had a treatment with that type of success rate for cancer, heart disease, or diabetes (and treating obesity can greatly reduce the risks for these diseases and improve remission rates), everyone would be taking advantage. So this begs the question: why aren't people with obesity getting the most effective treatment available?

Some may argue that it's "very dangerous," which would be a valid argument, if it were true. Sure, all surgical procedures and medical interventions come

---

[2] "Adult Obesity Facts," "Overweight & Obesity: Data & Statistics" section of Centers for Disease Control website, last modified May 17, 2022, https://www.cdc.gov/obesity/data/adult.html.
[3] "U.S. Obesity Rate Higher Than Ever," "Obesity in America" section of American Society for Metabolic and Bariatric Surgery website, published July 2021, https://asmbs.org/resources/obesity-in-america.
[4] ASMBS, "U.S. Obesity Rate."

with associated risks. However, as someone who has gone through weight loss surgery firsthand, I have some thoughts as to why more people aren't having bariatric surgery. If we push aside the risk factors, access to healthcare, and weight bias and discrimination (which are all certainly at play), there's one major reason I suspect people aren't getting the treatment.

I think what that boils down to is shame.

Unlike many other diseases, people who suffer from obesity are often blamed for their struggles. Being fat is seen as a moral failing. Those who don't embody society's ideals for thinness are extremely looked down upon. They are discriminated against, mocked, and ruthlessly told to just "do better." And once these people decide they might like to explore weight loss surgery, they are often met with comments like "Just try harder" or "Have you ever thought of dieting and exercising?" or (my favorite) "Wow, I can't believe you're taking the easy way out."

Ah yes, as if removing 85% of an organ, or bypassing it entirely, is easy. Though effective, weight loss surgery is anything *but* easy.

But unfortunately, society views weight loss surgery as a cop out. As a way for fat people to cheat the system, rather than cheating death. So many people are so afraid and ashamed of what others might think that they never reach out for help at all. Or they are conditioned to believe that they don't deserve help or don't even realize help exists for them.

So what do you do when you are struggling and need help but don't know where to turn? Or what happens when you have weight loss surgery and then have no follow-up support to lean on afterwards?

Because of the shame associated with bariatric surgery, so few people reach out for the support they need and deserve. Bariatric patients are historically an underserved population, and unfortunately, they are given very few resources for follow-up care and support. More often than not, this leaves them feeling overwhelmed, alone, and constantly worried they are going to "fail." The idea of failure for a bariatric patient is debilitating—not to mention the immense number of lifestyle and emotional changes they must go through in order to be successful. And while bariatric surgery is the number one most effective treatment for obesity, if the support and aftercare aren't sought out or provided, the likelihood of experiencing regain is high. Because if lifestyle changes aren't implemented long term, the weight can and will come back on. There are also many other nuances and factors that contribute to the sustainability of extreme weight loss results.

As both a registered dietitian and a weight loss surgery patient, I've experienced both the amazing wins as well as the overwhelming hurdles and pressures that bariatric surgery brings.

I've also experienced firsthand the major gaps in the medical system and how much we are lacking support, resources, and advocacy for bariatric surgery patients. I tried every diet, every program, saw every doctor and specialist, and was always left feeling defeated and worse off than when I started whatever fad program I was doing. I struggled my whole life. Not just from the weight, but from the shame, anxiety, and depression that came with it. I had thought about having weight loss surgery for years but kept pushing it off, too afraid of what others might think. Sometimes I wonder, *What would my life have been like had I taken the plunge sooner?*

For a long time, I was waiting to write about my journey until it was done. I didn't want to sit and put words to paper until I accomplished every goal and reached each milestone. But then, I realized that each time I hit a goal or achieved another accomplishment, I already had a new goal on my hands.

At first, I wanted to lose weight. So I did that. But I wasn't ready to write it down, because then I went to school to be a RD and wanted to wait until I had the credentials. But then I gained weight and certainly couldn't talk about a failed weight loss attempt; I mean, who would want to listen to that? So I set off to lose the weight again, this time with the help of weight loss surgery, but I couldn't write about it until I actually started losing weight.

After I lost 50 pounds, I decided it was best not to share until I'd lost at least 100 pounds. And then, once I hit these milestones, I didn't want to share my experiences until I had a business, because who would want to hear from someone without a brand? So I got my LLC and started coaching other people—both to help them and gain some experience before sharing with the rest of the world. Then I thought, *Nah, I have too much loose skin now. Best to wait until after I have plastics and am healed—then, THEN, I'll be done and ready to share my journey and knowledge with the world!* But no, because after that, I decided I still didn't look like the epitome of health and wanted to lose more weight, build muscle, and maybe even work toward some more athletic goals.

And then it hit me: nearly five years post weight loss surgery and three years into running my business, I realized this journey (both personally and professionally) does not end.

Your journey as a bariatric patient will never be done. You will never stop. You will never lose weight and hit the "finish line" and say, "Aha, now I am done. I am here and going nowhere else." There is also no end to providing support to those who are struggling and advocating for those whose stories so desperately need to be heard.

There is no finish line; you just keep going. Which direction you go is up to you. I've gone backwards before, and I've realized that going back to being obese, back to being miserable, back to disordered habits, back to hating and disappointing myself, is just no longer an option.

I may have dedicated my life to helping other women maintain their massive weight loss, empowering them with healthy habits and teaching food freedom as a way of doing so, but what I've really done is dedicate my own life to these principles too. I owe it to myself to keep going forward and to share everything I've learned about my journey, about postoperative care, and about food here with you.

Let me share with you my trials and triumphs. From morbidly obese to registered dietitian and all that happened in between. This is my life. My story. And it might sound a little like yours too.

Chapter 1
The Lifelong Battle

o·be·si·ty

/ōbēsədē/

noun

1. the state or condition of being very fat or overweight

"The girl was diagnosed with obesity at a young age."

2. the quality or fact of being very fat, in a way that is not healthy

"the problem of obesity among children"

Why Do People Even Have Weight Loss Surgery?

I am so glad you asked. Why would anyone opt for a life-changing permanent surgery when they could simply lose weight through traditional diet and exercise?

It's a valid question for sure; I'll give you that. The simplest answer I can provide is this: no one has weight loss surgery because it's their first choice. No one has weight loss surgery as a way to find a "loophole" for traditional diet and exercise. No one has surgery without trying everything under the sun first.

So while this question is a relevant and honest one, I think a better question to ask is this: "Why do some people try so hard to lose weight only to be unsuccessful at it?"

People have weight loss surgery not because they don't want to try to lose weight with traditional lifestyle changes (diet and exercise), but because they have tried the traditional route over and over again only to end up either right where they started or at an even higher weight than they were at the start of their last weight loss attempt. While there certainly are some folks who are able to lose an extreme amount of weight and maintain it without surgical or medical interventions, they tend to be the exception to the rule. Unfortunately, despite best efforts, that just isn't the case for the majority. The never-ending cycle of trying to overcome obesity is emotionally, physically, and mentally exhausting.

Obesity

Obesity is a disease. And that's not up for debate. I had a conversation with someone recently who stated, "I don't believe obesity is a disease." To which I laughed. It does not matter if you "believe" it to be a disease; the fact of the matter is it IS a disease.

As defined by WHO (World Health Organization), overweight and obesity are defined as "abnormal or excessive fat accumulation that presents a risk to health. A body mass index (BMI) over 25 is considered overweight, and over 30 is obese."[5] Now, let me be clear right off the bat: I think BMI as an indicator of health alone is complete and utter BS. BMI alone is an outdated metric that was created in the 1800s by a mathematician, not a physician. BMI doesn't take into account fat versus lean muscle percentage, nor does it tell you anything about one's health status. It was never meant to be an indicator of overall health, and BMI being used as an indicator of health is doubly harmful for BIPOC folks (Black, Indigenous, and People of Color) as it was never created with these folks in mind.

Luckily, the rest of the medical field is finally catching up. As of June 2023 the AMA (American Medical Association) has stated that "BMI is an imperfect measure because it does not directly assess body fat."[6] They have also conclud-

[5] "Obesity," "Health Topics" section of World Health Organization website, accessed July 14, 2023, https://www.who.int/health-topics/obesity#tab=tab_1.

[6] Sara Berg, "AMA: Use of BMI Alone Is an Imperfect Clinical Measure," American Medical Association website, published June 14, 2023, https://www.ama-assn.org/delivering-care/public-health/ama-

ed that the BMI classification system is misleading about the effects of body fat mass on mortality rates. The AMA's House of Delegates adopted a new policy recognizing the issues with BMI as a measurement due to the historical harm of relying on BMI and the use of BMI for racist exclusion.[7] Rather than assessing BMI alone as a diagnostic criteria, they are now saying that one's fat mass/visceral body fat, body composition, waist circumference, and metabolic and genetic factors should all be taken into consideration when diagnosing obesity. They also state that "relative body shape and composition heterogeneity across race and ethnic groups, sexes, genders and age-span is essential to consider when applying BMI as a measure of adiposity, and the use of BMI should not be used as a sole criterion to deny appropriate insurance reimbursement."[8] To this I say—well, it's about damn time!

I don't think the complexities of obesity are talked about or recognized enough. Obesity is a very complicated and multifaceted disease that affects the whole body and mind. According to the CDC (Center for Disease Control and Prevention), obesity is "a complex disease that occurs when an individual's weight is higher than what is considered healthy for his or her height. Many factors can contribute to excess weight gain, including eating patterns, physical activity levels, and sleep routines. Social determinants of health, genetics, and taking certain medications also play a role."[9] It is a disease that affects the whole person, and it's so much more than just the number on the scale.

In a nutshell, obesity results from chronic energy imbalance, meaning one's caloric intake exceeds what the person is able to expend based on their body's metabolic and physical functions.[10] For decades, researchers and health professionals have simplified the cure for obesity to being "calories in versus calories out," thus concluding that eating less and exercising more is the answer.

---

use-bmi-alone-imperfect-clinical-measure.

[7] Berg, "BMI."

[8] Berg, "BMI."

[9] "Causes of Obesity," "Overweight & Obesity: Obesity Basics" on CDC website, last updated March 21, 2022, https://www.cdc.gov/obesity/basics/causes.html.

[10] "Genes and Obesity," "Genomics & Precision Health" section of CDC website, last updated May 17, 2013, https://www.cdc.gov/genomics/resources/diseases/obesity/obesedit.htm.

They aren't necessarily wrong. In order to reduce body weight, you do need to be in a caloric deficit. But what we now know is that there are many barriers to that result, given the factors that contribute to the excessive intake and reduced expenditure in the first place. In the modern-day era we live in, the rise in obesity rates is largely linked to the reasons behind increased intake with reduced expenditure, known as an "obesogenic environment."[11]

Genetic factors play a very large role in obesity prevalence. While it's rare that people with obesity have one single gene that contributes to obesity, it's more common that a host of genetic factors drive up hunger, decrease satiety, and affect a wide variety of bodily functions and hormones. It's one of the reasons why even in an obesogenic environment, some struggle with obesity while others don't. [12]

Some people are genetically predisposed to be thinner while others are genetically predisposed to be larger. There are "naturally thin people" who don't have to work hard to be thin, they just are. Whereas "naturally larger people" have to work incredibly hard to be thin. There are also people who try to gain weight but can't. So why is it so hard to believe that some people could try and try to lose weight but can't?

Obesity, while a disease all on its own, also plays a huge role in other diseases. Obesity is a contributor to a host of other comorbidities, including (but not limited to) diseases such as type 2 diabetes (DM2), heart disease, high blood pressure, high cholesterol, gallstones, breathing and joint problems, and 13 different types of cancers, including breast cancer, thyroid cancer, liver cancer, pancreatic cancer, and meningioma.[13] People who struggle with obesity are at a much higher risk for many of these serious diseases than those at a "healthy" weight. (The word "healthy" is in quotations because weight alone doesn't determine one's overall health status.) In addition, people who struggle with obesity are also at a much higher risk for premature death and mental illness,

---

[11] CDC, "Genes and Obesity."
[12] CDC, "Genes and Obesity."
[13] "Obesity and Cancer," "Cancer: Risk Factors and Cancer" section of CDC website, last updated July 13, 2022, https://www.cdc.gov/cancer/obesity/index.htm.

such as clinical depression and anxiety.[14]

It's also important to bring to light the fact that so many diseases are precursors to obesity as well. Endocrine disorders such as PCOS, Cushing's syndrome, hypothyroidism, insulin resistance, and genetic disorders like Prader-Willi syndrome can all lead to obesity itself.

Childhood Obesity

Childhood obesity (the presence of obesity in children and adolescents) has been and continues to be a growing concern in the United States.

After compiling data on the prevalence of childhood obesity in the United States over the course of several years, the CDC published these findings in 2020:

- The prevalence of obesity was 19.7% and affected about 14.7 million children and adolescents.
- Obesity prevalence was 12.7% among 2-to-5-year-olds, 20.7% among 6- to 11-year-olds, and 22.2% among 12-to-19-year-olds. Childhood obesity is also more common among certain populations.
- Obesity prevalence was 26.2% among Hispanic children, 24.8% among non-Hispanic Black children, 16.6% among non-Hispanic White children, and 9.0% among non-Hispanic Asian children.
- Obesity-related conditions include high blood pressure, high cholesterol, type 2 diabetes, breathing problems such as asthma and sleep apnea, and joint problems.
- Obesity prevalence was 18.9% among children and adolescents aged 2-19 years in the lowest income group, 19.9% among those in the middle income group, and 10.9% among those in the highest income group.

---

[14] "Consequences of Obesity," "Overweight & Obesity: Obesity Basics" section of CDC website, last updated July 15, 2022, https://www.cdc.gov/obesity/basics/consequences.html.

- Obesity prevalence was lower in the highest income group among non-Hispanic Asian boys and Hispanic boys.
- Obesity prevalence was lower in the highest income group among non-Hispanic White girls, non-Hispanic Asian girls, and Hispanic girls. Obesity prevalence did not differ by income among non-Hispanic Black girls.[15]

Just like with adults, there are a lot of factors that contribute to childhood obesity, including lifestyle, genetics, environmental determinants, emotional factors, cultural nuances, and socioeconomic status. And don't think I'm skipping past the socioeconomic, cultural, and ethnic background factors, as these are very important and nuanced. We will circle back to this in Chapter 14.

Children who suffer from childhood obesity are also more likely to experience psychological problems such as anxiety and depression, low self-esteem, a lower self-reported quality of life, social problems such as bullying, and obesity in adulthood.[16] The psychological impacts obesity has on children and adolescents is also likely to carry over into adulthood.

I know many of you reading this might be sitting here thinking about your own childhoods, or perhaps you are even thinking about this through the lens of parenting your own children. While I'm not a parent, and have no idea what it is like to guide a child through these struggles, I know firsthand what it is like to be the child *with* these struggles.

My Childhood Obesity

I have struggled with obesity for as long as I can remember. When I was merely three, I started to peak on the growth charts. As a really young child, I was hyperaware of my body and my size. But it wasn't until I started school that I

[15] "Prevalence of Childhood Obesity in the United States," "Overweight & Obesity: Data & Statistics: Childhood Obesity Facts" section of CDC website, last updated May 17, 2022, https://www.cdc.gov/obesity/data/childhood.html.
[16] CDC, "Consequences of Obesity."

was able to recognize how different I was from other kids. My very first memory of being made fun of for my weight was when I was about six. My next-door neighbor, who was my age, used to come over before and after school; and one day, I remember her making fun of me for being fat. I think it was the first time I can recall feeling ashamed of my body. I wish it was also the last. But I suppose if feeling shame and disgust toward my own body never happened, I wouldn't be here writing this book for you, would I?

Did you know that your most influential programming is formed in your subconscious by the age of seven?[17] In other words, the things we believe about ourselves are formed by the age of seven, based on all the things said to and around us, as well as our lived and perceived experiences.

When I think about this, it makes a lot of sense. It explains why I was always so "shy" growing up. For the first 25 years of my life, I believed I was an introvert. The truth is, I'm not actually an introvert; I just *believed* I was, because people would say, "Oh Jamie is just so shy" and "Jamie is so quiet." Which I was. But it's not because I *am* quiet or shy; it's because the shame and fear I felt from a young age shaped me into that mold. And with each shameful experience, I got a little quieter and a little more reserved. Almost as a defense. If they didn't see or hear me, they couldn't say anything bad about me, could they? Turns out they could, and they still did.

It's wild how the most hurtful experiences are the ones that stay with you the longest. I've had a lot of shitty things said to me over the years, particularly about my weight. But I think the hardest one for me to remember is what my grandmother said to me when I was eight years old.

"Jamie," she said, as she piled another serving of mac and cheese onto my plate, "You really need to do something about your weight. If you don't lose

---

[17] Kyndall Watkins, "Reprogram Your Sub Conscience Mind for Success," Eastern Carolina University's Campus Recreation & Wellness website, published October 10, 2019, https://crw.ecu.edu/2019/10/10/if-you-feel-like-giving-up/#:~:text=Beginning%20from%20the%20time%20that,shows%20and%20movies%20you%20watched.

weight, boys will never like you when you're older."

"I know, Nana," I said. "I'm trying. I know I need to lose a few pounds."

"A few?" She snorted. "You need to lose forty pounds, at least."

I went home that night and cried when I told my mother what her mother said to me. Naturally, my mom lost it on my grandmother, so my grandmother made it a point to yell at me the next time I saw her. "Look at you, always running and telling your mom. You're so *sensitive*," she said.

That insult has been slung in my face my whole life. *Sensitive*. God, I hate that word. My number one piece of advice for anyone who ever comes into contact with a child is to make sure you never tell them they are "too sensitive" when they express their feelings. Because do you know what that does? It signals to them that their feelings are bad. That their feelings are invalid. That they shouldn't feel the things that they feel. What makes it one thousand times worse is that those feelings I felt in those moments were a direct result of the things that were said to me. And those suppressed feelings further fed the toxic relationship I had with food, as I continually stuffed my feelings down with the very thing that was causing the "problem" in the first place.

When you perceive your own feelings as bad, you do your best not to feel them. You do your best to ignore them. To stuff them down with whatever means possible. You cover them up as best you can. You replace them with the feelings you know are seen as "good" or that bring you joy—kind of like that feeling I would get when I would eat the foods I loved. Why feel those icky, gross emotions when I could cover it up with some cookies and milk?

I'm not blaming anyone for my struggles with my weight and my relationship with food. But there are environmental and genetic components that contribute to eating disorders too. So while it's not directly any one person's fault, all I'm saying is being told by my own family, who also struggled with their own weight and ate their feelings, that I needed to be on a diet at eight years old certainly didn't help matters.

Because at eight, I had no business even thinking about diets. I shouldn't have been so aware of my body by the age of four either. I shouldn't have been shamed at every angle for the foods I ate or how I ate them. These weren't conversations that should have been had in front of me or around me. But they were.

I don't have all the solutions to childhood obesity, and as I said before, I have no idea what it's like to raise a child who struggles. But I can tell you this much: don't have these conversations with them or around them. You aren't doing them any favors, and you certainly aren't saving them from obesity as an adult.

Set Point Theory

I believe set point theory is one of the reasons why children with obesity often become adults with obesity. I also believe it's why so many adults try to lose weight only to gain it back. On top of every factor previously mentioned, set point theory, I believe, plays a big role.

Set point theory states that there are biological regulators and factors that determine your body's weight.[18] Some scientists and obesity specialists don't believe in set point, hence it just being a theory thus far. There is still a lot we don't know about this theory. While lots of factors determine one's weight, and I don't think it is a finalized determinant of one's weight outcomes, I do think there is some validity to it.

Biologically, our bodies are designed and engineered to keep us alive. Homeostasis, by definition, is the state at which our body is at balance and maintains equilibrium. There are physiologic processes within our bodies, made up of

[18] "What is Set Point Weight?," "Weight Loss & Obesity: Reference" section of WebMD.com, last updated May 21, 2023, https://www.webmd.com/obesity/what-is-set-point-weight.

checks-and-balances systems, which help our bodies maintain equilibrium and ultimately keep us alive. Drastic changes disrupt homeostasis and these checks-and-balances systems, and your body is biologically driven to try to get you back to your previous state. In other words, if you lose a significant amount of weight, it signals to your body that something is "wrong." And in an effort to "protect" you, your body will try to get your body back to its original state.

Our bodies like to be at a higher weight. This is because weight, and having enough body fat on our bodies, keeps us alive. It is protective and keeps us safe. Back in our prehistoric era, our ancestors didn't always know where their next meal was coming from. Food was often scarce. However, when you are in a state of famine, you don't just drop dead. Our bodies evolved to keep us alive and function even when we are not continually eating. Our bodies have the ability to pull from our fat stores to use them as energy, even in long periods of time between meals. Because of this, our bodies *like* having extra weight on us. And if you lose a significant amount of weight, your body will do its best to get you back to your set point—that higher, stable weight you once had—as a way to protect you.

Thanks, body! Love that you care so much about us! BUT the thing is, we are no longer in prehistoric caveman times. We live in modern times, where food is (for the most part) more readily and abundantly available. We live in a world where *most* grocery stores are stocked and there are fast food joints and convenience stores on every corner. Now, that's not to ignore the fact that some places are still deemed as food deserts, and food scarcity and accessibility are still major issues in certain places and for different demographics. Whether or not everyone has access to these things is a totally different (and important) conversation. But for you and me (and for the sake of this point), I think it's safe to say that it's important to realize the distinction between prehistoric times versus the modern world we live in today.

Why? Because our biological evolution has not caught up with societal evolution, our bodies are still working to protect us and keep the weight on, even though food is no longer scarce—which helps to explain why, even after someone has lost a lot of weight, it's often so hard to keep it off despite best efforts. Although there is some research to support that having weight loss surgery *may* help adjust someone's set point weight to a lower range, there is still a lot about set point theory that we don't know.[19]

An example of how set point theory might make sense in "real life" might look a little something like this: Let's imagine we have two people.

- **Person #1:** A 5'4" female who is 145 pounds, who has never dieted in her life, and who does not struggle to maintain her 145-pound weight. She can eat upwards of 2500 calories per day with little effect on her weight. She also does not restrict calories or certain types of foods, and generally feels very satisfied at meal and snack times. Other than general activity (walking, being active, etc.), she does not regularly exercise.
- **Person #2:** A 5'4" female who is 145 lbs, who has dieted most of her life, has lost 100+ pounds in the last three years, and has to work very hard to maintain her weight. She eats approximately 1300 calories per day, is very mindful of both her calorie intake and food quality intake, and often feels hungry throughout the day. She goes to the gym 4–5 times per week and takes long walks regularly. If she goes up on her calories, or decreases her activity, she will very quickly and easily regain the weight she spent so many years losing.

We see this all the time. And granted, there are other factors at play (such as hormones, genetics, environmental factors, etc.), but it's not unusual for someone who has never struggled with their weight to be able to maintain their weight with little effort, whilst someone of the same body size and composition who has lost a significant amount of weight struggles so hard to stay there. While the

[19] Malini Ghoshal, "What You Need to Know about Set Point Theory," "Health" section of Healthline.com, https://www.healthline.com/health/set-point-theory#changing-a-set-point.

first person is able to more easily metabolize their food, the second person will need to burn significantly more calories in order to achieve the same outcomes.

There certainly are lots of ways for person #2 to combat these things (for example: building muscle, having additional medication support, etc.), so please don't read this and think you are doomed to struggle forever, but it is important to take note of the additional struggles someone with lifelong obesity will likely have as opposed to someone who hasn't struggled with it.

Things to Consider and Treatments for Obesity

Now, fear not, my friends! I don't want you to read this and think, *Great, I was an overweight kid, and I'm now an overweight adult; and now, because of set point theory, I'm destined to always be overweight no matter what.*

I can see how you might draw that conclusion, but it's not quite true. There's more to consider. Thankfully, we do have control over reducing our body weight. With a combination of lifestyle changes, healthy habits, mindset shifts, self-care routines, and medical interventions—including combinations of surgical interventions and medication—weight loss and sustained weight loss is absolutely possible and achievable.

But I think one of the biggest things to consider is that obesity is a chronic disease, meaning it's lifelong. Did you know that fat cells are the only cells within our body that can't die? I know, how rude! While your fat cells will deplete with weight loss, they are still there, ready to plump back up at any time, thanks to set point theory. And even depleted fat cells are metabolically active, meaning they require energy. So someone who lost a lot of weight is likely to still require more energy and have a larger appetite than someone of the same weight who did not go through major weight loss, and that's because their metabolic needs are still greater to support their body.

All of that being said, there are effective treatments for obesity, but even if someone loses weight and is no longer considered "obese" or "overweight," they still will have to manage that chronic disease forever, even after they lose the weight. It's a lifelong condition to be managed.

And it's not your fault. If you have struggled over and over, time and time again, to lose weight and keep it off but haven't been "successful," you are not alone. And more importantly, you are not a failure. There is hope, and it is NEVER too late to take control of your life, your health, and overcome your obesity. It's a disease, not a moral failing or an indication of your character. And if you'd like to overcome it and break through the never-ending cycle, I'd like to help you by sharing all the treatment options, things to consider, and nuances that others may not have talked to you about. There's a lot to go through, but I hope you'll stick around.

Bite-Sized Recap

- People have weight loss surgery not because they don't want to try to lose weight with traditional lifestyle changes (diet and exercise), but because they have tried the traditional route over and over again, only to end up either right where they started or at an even higher weight than at the start of their last weight loss attempt.
- Obesity is a complex, multifaceted, multilayered disease that involves genetic, environmental, emotional, psychological, cultural, and socio-economic components.
- BMI (body mass index) is not a good indicator of one's overall health nor should it be used to evaluate one's health status.
- Childhood obesity is a growing concern that links heavily to obesity in adulthood.
- Set point theory may help us understand why it is often so hard for individuals with lifelong obesity to lose weight and maintain it.

For journal prompts and resources related to this chapter, be sure to head to www.thesleeveddietitian.com/easy.

Chapter 2
Bariatric Surgery

bar·iat·rics

/ber-ē-a-triks/

plural in form but singular in construction

noun

1. The branch of medicine that deals with the treatment of obesity.

"Bariatrics is an evolving and changing field."

My Experience with Bariatric Surgery

I wish I could recall the first time I learned what bariatric surgery was, but I can't. But what I will say is it was probably on my radar a lot sooner in life than one might expect.

While I don't remember where I first learned about surgery, what I do remember is being 14, a freshman in high school, and absolutely begging my mom to let me get the lap band procedure.

I've always been the type of person that when my mind is set on something, I can't get the idea out of my head. I hyperfixate on it and learn all I can about it. I remember I had researched all I could on weight loss surgery. I remember printing out articles, gathering information, and going as far as signing up for information seminars (unbeknownst to my mother) at local weight loss surgery centers.

In my 14-year-old head, I was convinced that if I presented my mom with all the facts, took out all the guesswork by being proactive and signing myself up for the seminars, and could just prove to her that this was the answer to all my problems, she simply could not say no.

Turns out she could. And she did.

"You're not getting weight loss surgery," she said.

Naturally, I argued and continued to try and convince her. Eventually I stopped asking when I realized she wasn't going to be persuaded.

In retrospect, I'm really grateful she told me no. Fourteen-year-old Jamie still had a lot to learn and to go through before she would be ready for weight loss surgery. While pediatric bariatric procedures are an option (pediatric, referring to weight loss surgeries in adolescents under 21 years old), an option I am in favor of for the right person, it wouldn't have been the right option for me, no matter how much I thought it was at the time.

I had all but abandoned the idea of surgery for years after that. And I'm even a bit embarrassed to admit that in my late teens and very early twenties, as I had embarked on one of my many weight loss attempts, I had actually started to look down upon weight loss surgery.

During this era in my life, I was truly in the depths of toxic diet culture. I was losing weight in some pretty unhealthy ways, although at the time, I thought I was doing everything "right." I was doing it "naturally." And if I was working my ass off to do things "right," why shouldn't everyone? Ah yes, my friends, at one time I too was of the mindset that bariatric surgery was somehow "wrong." That people who chose it simply just weren't trying hard enough. And if I could buck up and try harder, why couldn't everyone else?

Let's just say 19-year-old Jamie had about as much to learn as 14-year-old Jamie. And boy did she eat her own words down the line, because fast-forward five years, I found myself at the ripe old age of 24, sitting at my first consultation with my bariatric surgeon.

After losing and regaining 70 pounds, and going through hell and back with disordered eating, PCOS symptoms, and everything in between, I finally had realized there was no pride in doing it the "natural" way. At least not for me. Not if it didn't allow me to be the healthiest version of me, mentally or physically.

Over five years later, and I can report back to you all that bariatric surgery was the best decision I ever could have made for myself. It was hard, really hard actually, much harder than I anticipated. It hasn't been a straight path or a linear road. There have been bumps along the way, but overall, my experience with weight loss surgery has been amazing. It changed my life for the better, in so many ways, and I'll never stop being grateful for the second chance at life that it gave me.

What Does "Bariatric" Mean?

By definition, "bariatrics" is the branch of medicine that deals with the study and treatment of obesity. It is an umbrella term that includes a multitude of medical interventions to treat and manage the disease of obesity, and by default, to manage and treat the comorbidities that coincide with obesity. Some examples of comorbidities include sleep apnea, high blood pressure, type 2 diabetes, high cholesterol, and heart disease—all diseases that have the potential to be brought on or worsened by obesity, which is why treating obesity often has a domino effect on one's health.

The two main medical interventions that are currently available to treat obesity include medication and surgical interventions. A bit later, I'm going to dive into the different medication management options and how those treatments alone, or in conjunction with surgery, can be optimal for long-term weight loss success. But for now, I'm going to break down the different bariatric surgical procedures: what they do, how they work, and what lifestyle changes need to be made before and after. I'm also going to explain to you WHY these lifestyle changes need to be implemented.

There are 2 branches of medical interventions for obesity treatment

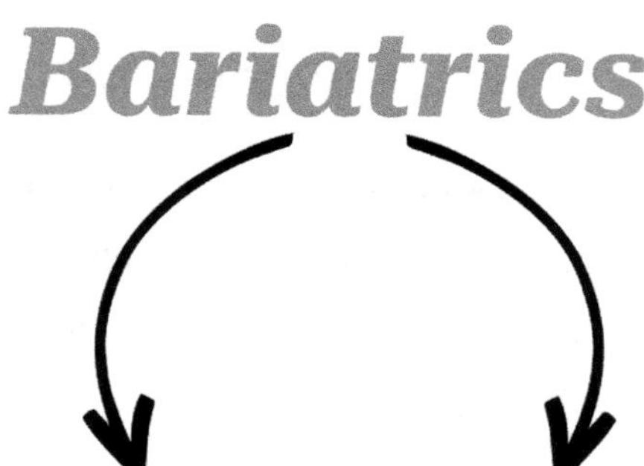

Medication Management

Pharmaceutical Options

- Phentermine (Suprenza)
- Orlistat (Alli)
- Phentermine-Topiramate (Qsymia)
- Bupropion/Naltrexone (Contrave)
- Liraglutide/GLP-1 (Sazenda/Victoza)
- Dulaglutide (Trulicity)
- Semaglutide/ GLP-1 (Ozempic/ Wegovy)
- Tirzepatide / GLP-1 & GIP (Mounjaro)

Surgical Interventions

Surgical Options

- Adjustable Gastric Banding
- Gastric Balloon
- Roux - En - Y Gastric Bypass
- Mini-Gastric Bypass or One Anastomosis Gastric Bypass
- Vertical Sleeve Gastrectomy
- Duodenal Switch
- SADI-S
- Revisional Surgeries

Diagram showing the two branches of medical interventions for treating obesity. The image title reads "Bariatrics" and has two downward pointing arrows. On the left side of the image, medical management and pharmaceutical options are listed as follows: phentermine (Suprenza), orlistat (Alli), phentermine-topiramate (Qsymia), bupropion/naltrexone (Contrave), liraglutide/GLP-1 (Sazenda/Victoza), dulaglutide (Trulicity), semaglutide/ GLP-1 (Ozempic/ Wegovy), tirzepatide/GLP-1 & GIP (Mounjaro)

On the right side of the image, surgical interventions and options listed as follows: adjustable gastric banding, gastric balloon, Roux-en-Y gastric bypass, mini-gastric bypass or one anastomosis gastric bypass, vertical sleeve gastrectomy, duodenal switch, SADI-S, revisional surgeries

The Types of Surgeries Available

There are so many different types of bariatric surgeries, and as the science and understanding of bariatrics keeps expanding, new improvements to these surgical procedures continue to advance. Some of the most common surgeries include adjustable gastric band (also referred to as the lap band or AGB), the gastric balloon, Roux-en-Y gastric bypass (RYGB or RNY), one anastomosis gastric bypass (OAGB, also sometimes referred to as "mini-gastric bypass" or mini GBP), vertical sleeve gastrectomy (VSG), duodenal switch (DS), and the single anastomosis duodenal switch with sleeve gastrectomy (SADI-S). There are additional surgery types and other variations of the above procedures, including revision surgeries, but for the purposes of this chapter, we will be focusing on these most commonly recommended surgeries.

In addition to all of the surgeries available, there are both metabolic and non-metabolic procedures as well as malabsorptive and non-malabsorptive procedures.

The term "metabolic" refers to one's metabolism. By definition, metabolism is the process by which the body changes food and drink into energy. During this process, calories in food and drinks mix with oxygen to make the energy the body needs.[20] Your metabolism is responsible for converting calories to energy as well as burning this energy. There are so many chemical reactions and hormones involved in one's metabolism.

I like to tell my clients that our bodies are so cool, because their only job is to keep us safe and alive. It's really so amazing that our internal systems, cells, organs, and hormones all "speak" to one another in order to keep our bodies functioning and in balance. There are so many different hormones within our body that keep us alive, and they require what's described as "feedback loops" to provide our systems with homeostasis.

The fundus of the stomach (the bottom portion of the stomach), is where the hormone called **ghrelin** is produced. Ghrelin is known as the "hunger hormone." Normally, when we eat, ghrelin signals to our brain that we are hungry. This hunger drives us to eat. As we eat, hormones from our intestines are re-

---

20 "Metabolism and Weight Loss: How You Burn Calories," "Healthy Lifestyle: Weight Loss" section of Mayo Clinic website, last updated October 8, 2022, https://www.mayoclinic.org/healthy-lifestyle/weight-loss/in-depth/metabolism/art-20046508#:~:text=Metabolism%20is%20the%20process%20by,the%20energy%20the%20body%20needs.

leased. These hormones are known as **gastric inhibitory polypeptide (GIP)** and **glucagon-like peptide-1 (GLP-1)**, which are the two primary incretin hormones "secreted from the intestine on ingestion of glucose or nutrients to stimulate insulin secretion from pancreatic β cells."[21]

Once insulin is released from the pancreas, it allows the sugar in our bloodstream to be taken into our cells to be used as energy. As we eat and our bodies use the food for energy, **leptin**—also known as the "satiety" hormone—is secreted from your adipose tissue (fat cells) to signal to your body that you are full and satisfied and no longer need to continue eating. Once leptin is secreted, it turns off the ghrelin in your stomach.

Now, typically, for people who don't struggle with obesity or hormonal imbalances, these homeostatic systems work beautifully. However, obesity is a disease. A complex and multifaceted disease with many hormonal, genetic, emotional, and environmental components to it (and yes, I'm going to keep reiterating this, just to make sure it sinks in). But with that being said, people who struggle with obesity often are much hungrier and less satiated when eating for a multitude of reasons, which further contributes to their struggles.

Because of this, weight loss surgeries that have metabolic effects can be extremely impactful for people who have struggled with obesity. Beyond just supporting people with portion control, many bariatric surgeries are true metabolic surgeries because they have the ability to change one's hormonal makeup through the alteration of the anatomy.

In addition to metabolic versus non-metabolic procedures, there are also what's called malabsorptive procedures. All of the malabsorptive procedures are inherently metabolic ones as well. By definition, malabsorption prevents the body from effectively absorbing nutrients from your food.[22] For the meta-

[21] Yutaka Seino et al., "GIP and GLP-1, the Two Incretin Hormones: Similarities and Differences," *Journal of Diabetes Investigation* 1, no 1–2 (April 2022): 8–23, https://pubmed.ncbi.nlm.nih.gov/24843404/,
[22] "Malabsorption," "Health Library: Diseases & Conditions" section of Cleveland Clinic website, last updated April 6, 2022, https://my.clevelandclinic.org/health/diseases/22722-malabsorption.

bolic procedures that have this additional malabsorptive component, there is usually a more significant weight loss as a result, since not all of the calories and nutrients the patient consumes will be absorbed, minimizing the person's calorie intake even further.

That said, there are other considerations to take into consideration, which we will dive into.

Non-Metabolic Procedures: The Adjustable Gastric Band (AGB) and Gastric Balloon

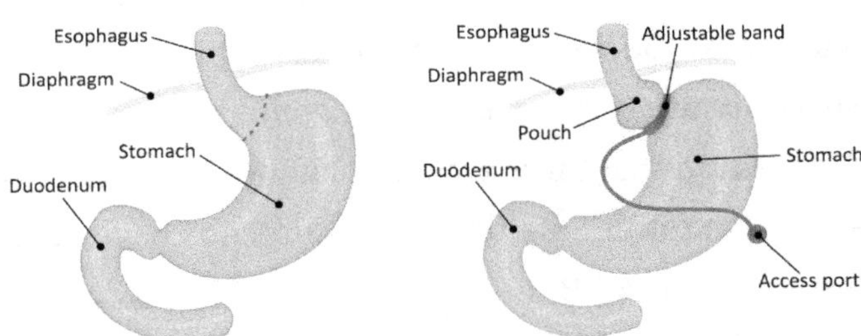

Anatomical depiction of a stomach undergoing the adjustable gastric band procedure. An adjustable band is placed near the top of the stomach, and an access port is accessible outside the body for modifications.

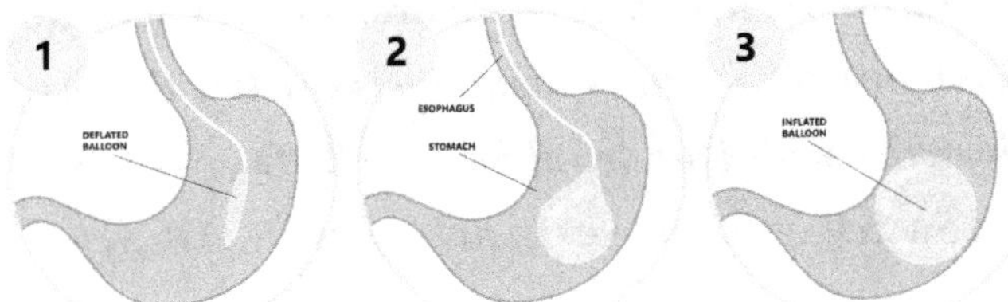

Anatomical depiction of a stomach undergoing the intragastric balloon procedure. A deflated balloon is threaded down the esophagus to the middle of the stomach, where it is then inflated.

These are the bariatric procedures that do not alter one's metabolic or hormonal makeup. These procedures are primarily used for portion control to support people in achieving weight loss.

The AGB and gastric balloon are often seen as less invasive, since they are the only bariatric procedures that are not permanent. With the AGB, an adjustable band is placed around the opening of the stomach and fluid is added through an access port, making the band tighter or looser (depending on how much fluid is added or taken away), which creates more or less restriction. With the gastric balloon, a temporary device (a deflated "balloon") is placed into the patient's stomach and then inflated. With the balloon filling the stomach space, the patient feels fuller quicker and can restrict their portion size, which (alongside lifestyle changes) usually results in less calorie intake and greater weight loss results.

The AGB can stay in place long term, as long as there are no complications, whereas the gastric balloon must be removed, typically within six months. While these surgeries are reversible, they may not result in as great of weight loss for the main reason that there are no metabolic changes or malabsorptive effects. It's also important to note that many surgeons have personally chosen to no longer perform the AGB due to limited weight loss and complications. That doesn't mean these procedures can't be reasonable options for the right patients. Some people, particularly lower BMI patients, may do well with these surgeries in both the long and short terms.

Metabolic Procedures: Vertical Sleeve Gastrectomy (VSG), Roux-en-Y Gastric Bypass (RYGB or RNY), One Anastomosis Gastric Bypass (OAGB), Biliopancreatic Diversion with Duodenal Switch (BPD or DS), & Single Anastomosis Duodenal Switch with Sleeve Gastrectomy (SADI-S)

The vertical sleeve gastrectomy (VSG) has become one of the most common bariatric surgeries performed in the US and worldwide.[23] With VSG, approx-

[23] Kristina H. Lewis et al., "Comparative Effectiveness of Vertical Sleeve Gastrectomy vs. Roux en Y Gastric Bypass for Diabetes Treatment: A Claims-Based Cohort Study," *Annals of Surgery* 273, no. 5 (May 2021), 940–948, "https://www.ncbi.nlm.nih.gov/pmc/articles/PMC7402414/#:~:text=Vertical%20Sleeve%20Gastrectomy%20(VSG)%20has,the%20United%20States%20and%20worldwide.&-text=Little%20over%20a%20decade%20ago,Y%20Gastric%20Bypass%20(RYGB).

imately 80-85% of the stomach is removed, including the fundus of the stomach, where ghrelin is produced. The remaining stomach size and shape is com parable to that of a banana.[24] This removal of a portion of the stomach, along with the hormone ghrelin, is what categorizes it as a metabolic procedure. With VSG, malabsorption isn't a factor. It's said to be one of the "simpler" procedures and doesn't take as long to perform as some of the other more involved procedures, making it an ideal option for many patients, especially those who may be at higher medical risk for undergoing surgery.[25]

Vertical Sleeve Gastrectomy

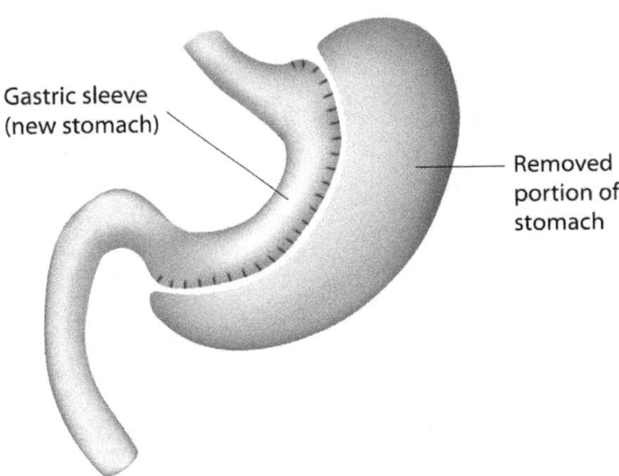

Anatomical depiction of a stomach undergoing the vertical sleeve gastrectomy procedure. A large portion of the stomach (approximately 85%) is removed, and the remainder of the stomach is internally stitched up creating a small stomach pouch that resembles the shape of a banana.

Roux-en-Y Gastric bypass (RYGB or RNY) is the bariatric surgery that has been around the longest, and has now been performed for more than 50 years, with the laparoscopic approach being refined since 1993.[26] During the RNY procedure, a small pouch is created at the top of the stomach and is directly attached to the small intestines, bypassing the original stomach completely. The new stomach, or "pouch," is typically the size of an egg or a golf ball.

---

[24] "Bariatric Surgery Procedures," Patient Learning Center, Public Education Committee of the ASMBS, last updated May 2021, https://asmbs.org/patients/bariatric-surgery-procedures.
[25] ASMBS, "Bariatric Surgery Procedures."
[26] ASMBS, "Bariatric Surgery Procedures."

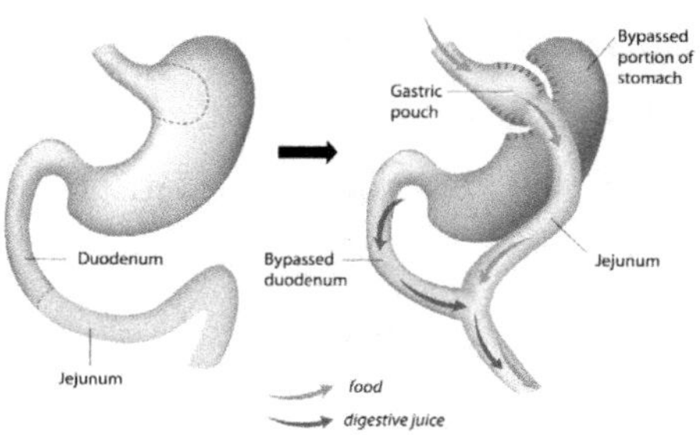

Anatomical depiction of a stomach undergoing the Roux -en-Y gastric bypass procedure. A gastric pouch is created at the top portion of the stomach. The bottom portion of the new pouch is attached to the jejunum, bypassing the original stomach and duodenum.

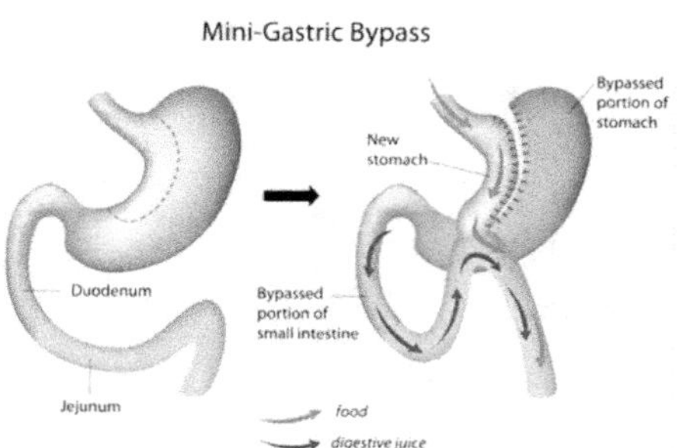

Anatomical depiction of a stomach undergoing the one anastomosis gastric bypass or mini-gastric bypass procedure. A new stomach pouch is created that is larger in size than the traditional gastric bypass pouch but smaller in size than the vertical sleeve gastrectomy pouch, and the bottom of the pouch is attached to the jejunum, bypassing the stomach.

RNY works in several ways. The golf-ball-sized pouch helps the patient consume fewer calories. Additionally, none of the food that is consumed comes into contact with the first part of the small intestine, which results in decreased absorption.[27] During the RNY procedure, "the small intestine is then divided to separate the upper and lower parts, known as the duodenum and the jejunum. The new stomach pouch is attached to the lower portion of the small intestine, or jejunum, while the upper portion of the small intestine, or duodenum, is connected further down the small intestine."[28]

Similarly, the one anastomosis gastric bypass (OAGB, or more commonly known as the "mini" gastric bypass) reduces the stomach size; however, the new pouch created with the OAGB is a bit larger. And "rather than dividing

[27] ASMBS, "Bariatric Surgery Procedures."
[28] Bryee Shepard, "Mini-Gastric Bypass vs. RNY Gastric Bypass," Pre Surgery section of Barilife.com, accessed July 24, 2023, https://www.barilife.com/blog/mini-gastric-bypass/.

the small intestine, the new stomach pouch is attached directly to the jejunum."[29] Since there is only one new connection made, versus two, during this procedure, it is simplified and results in a shorter operative time.

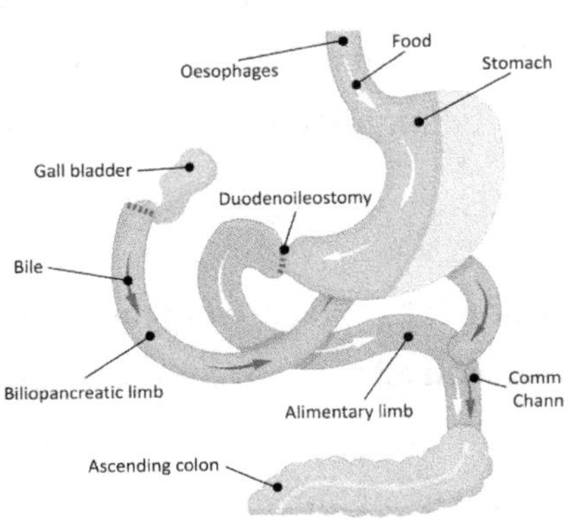

Anatomical depiction of a stomach undergoing the biliopancreatic diversion with a duodenal switch procedure. A small tube-shaped stomach pouch is created, then the first portion of the small intestine is separated from the stomach, and last, a part of the small intestine is brought up and connected to the outlet of the new stomach, creating two surgical bowel connections.

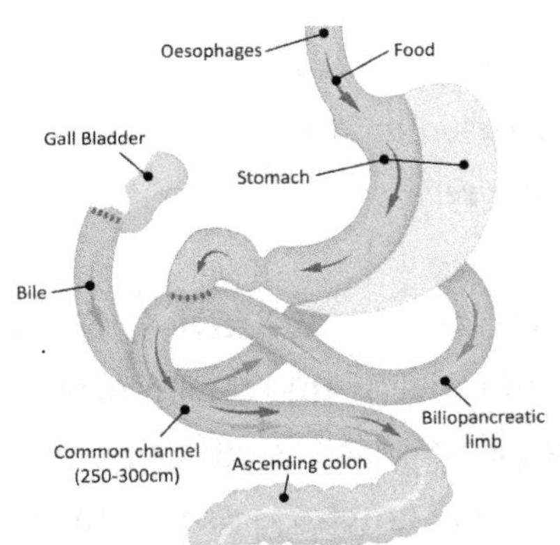

Anatomical depiction of a stomach undergoing the SADI-S procedure. The SADI-S procedure is very similar to that depicted in Image 8, the difference being that there is no duodenal switch implemented here.

The biliopancreatic diversion with duodenal switch (DS) procedure is somewhat of a "combination" of VSG and RNY (well, sort of). With DS, a smaller stomach is created in a similar fashion as with VSG. This procedure begins with the creation of a small tube-shaped stomach (like the remaining stomach after VSG). Following the creation of this sleeve-like stomach, the first portion of the small intestine is separated from the stomach, which makes it similar to RNY, where the first section of the small intestine is not used.[30] After that, a part of the small intestine is brought up and connected to the outlet of the new stomach, so that when the person eats, the food goes through the sleeve-

[29] Shepard, "Mini-Gastric Bypass."
[30] ASMBS, "Bariatric Surgery Procedures."

like-pouch stomach and then enters into the latter part of the small intestine.[31]

Similarly, the single anastomosis duodenal switch with sleeve gastrectomy (SADI-S) is performed this way as well, except this procedure is said to be "simpler" than the original DS since there is only one surgical bowel connection as opposed to two. This makes the length of the surgical procedure shorter and thus safer for many patients. It is the most recent bariatric procedure to be endorsed by the ASMBS and is said to be highly effective for long-term weight loss results.[32]

With RNY, DS, and the SADI-S, malabsorption takes place, whereas with VSG, there is minimal (if any) malabsorption. But with all three of these procedures, the original stomach is either removed or bypassed, removing or bypassing the area where ghrelin is produced, making them all metabolic procedures.

Who Qualifies for Weight Loss Surgery?

After reading about all the different surgeries, you might be wondering, *How do I get one of these surgeries? Who qualifies*? Well, thanks to infamous shows like *My 600-lb Life*, our society seems to have this misconception that one must be bedbound due to their weight in order to qualify for weight loss surgery. I'm excited to share that that is luckily not the case.

Each bariatric surgery program has slightly different requirements, as do various insurance companies. But generally speaking, in order to qualify for surgery, you must either have a BMI of 35 or greater without the presence of co-morbidities or have a BMI of 30–35 with comorbidities such as type 2 diabetes and demonstrate that you have been unable to achieve substantial or durable weight loss or co-morbidity improvement using nonsurgical methods.[33] Co-morbidities are typically identified as having high blood pressure, high cholesterol, type 2 diabetes, cardiovascular diseases and/or sleep apnea.

---

[31] ASMBS, "Bariatric Surgery Procedures."

[32] ASMBS, "Bariatric Surgery Procedures."

[33] "Who Is a Candidate for Bariatric Surgery?" "Patient Learning Center" on ASMBS website, accessed July 14, 2023, https://asmbs.org/patients/who-is-a-candidate-for-bariatric-surgery.

Now remember, we could spend all day discussing why BMI is a garbage indicator of health, but when strictly looking at classes of obesity alone, if you fall into one of these categories, you might qualify.

If you're sitting here thinking about your own BMI and going, *Damn, I didn't realize that was me,* welcome to the club, my friend. So many people are largely offended when they learn and realize that they qualify for surgery. In our later chapters, I'm going to get into some of the reasons why so few people realize they qualify and why so many people underutilize bariatric surgery.

There's a lot more that goes into receiving bariatric surgery than BMI alone, of course. Like I mentioned, each surgical center and insurance company has their own set of requirements in order to get clearance for surgery. On average, it takes anywhere from three to six months from your first surgical consult to receiving your surgery date. Most programs and insurance companies will require you to attend an information seminar, schedule an initial consult, and complete a panel of extensive blood work, a pulmonary evaluation, an EKG, an endoscopy, a sleep study (if your neck circumference is >40cm), a PCP pre-op evaluation, a psychological evaluation, and anywhere from three to six months of dietitian visits. This is to make sure that you are a good candidate for surgery and are fully educated and prepared to make all the lifestyle, dietary, and habit changes necessary to have a safe and successful surgery.

Lifestyle Changes Pre- and Post-Op

As I said before, our bodies are just SO smart. Even after undergoing a metabolic procedure, over time, our bodies learn to adapt and begin producing ghrelin again, making bariatric patients regain their hunger signals. This is, once again, where homeostasis kicks in.

Usually around 18 months post-op is when bariatric patients typically start to experience that hunger sensation again (assuming their hunger sensation was minimized after surgery, as some patients do still report hunger immediately after). The first 12–18 months post weight loss surgery is often referred to as the "honeymoon phase" for this exact reason. In that first 12–18 months, most will report not feeling intense hunger or cravings (although some might still experience this). Also in those first 12–18 months is when restriction is the tightest—meaning, you are full relatively quickly and aren't able to eat very much at one time. It's a double whammy of extreme portion control combined with the metabolic effects I mentioned above. This is why the "rules" that need to be followed after weight loss surgery are so important, which I will get into in Chapter 9.

This journey is more than just following a diet. With your anatomy being changed, there are a lot of unique rules that need to be followed after surgery. Not just for weight loss and long-term weight maintenance, but for safety. Which is why bariatric surgery comes with its own unique set of rules.

One of the things that so many people don't realize is that when you have bariatric surgery, a lot of the habits you have to change are more than just your nutritional habits. There are so many changes physically, mentally, and emotionally that go into a bariatric journey. Diet and food is really just one piece of the puzzle.

When you have weight loss surgery, you are physically changing your anatomy. With that comes a different set of "rules," for lack of a better term, that need to be followed. These rules have little to nothing to do with weight loss or the rate of weight loss, but everything to do with your safety and your health. I dive into some of these rules and lifestyle changes later in the book.

However, despite these "rules" and how far we've come around body positivity and inclusivity, there's still a lot of weight stigma and bias in the world (especially when you look through the lens of social media).

It's important, whether you are opting for surgery or are a practitioner in this field, to understand the biases that still exist and make sure you are doing the work to not perpetuate these stigmas, consciously or subconsciously.

Bite-Sized Recap

- Bariatrics is the branch of medicine that deals with the study and treatment of obesity. It is an umbrella term that includes a multitude of medical interventions to treat and manage the disease of obesity, and by default, to manage and treat the comorbidities that coincide with obesity. Some examples of comorbidities include sleep apnea, high blood pressure, type 2 diabetes, high cholesterol, and heart disease—all of which have the potential to be brought on or worsened by obesity, which is why treating obesity often has a domino effect on one's health.
- The two main medical interventions that are currently available to treat obesity include medication and surgical interventions.
- The most common surgeries include adjustable gastric band (also referred to as the lap band or AGB), the gastric balloon, Roux-en-Y gastric bypass (RYGB or RNY), one anastomosis gastric bypass (OAGB, often called "mini-gastric bypass"), vertical sleeve gastrectomy (VSG), duodenal switch (DS), and the single anastomosis duodenal switch with sleeve gastrectomy (SADI-S).
- There are both metabolic and non-metabolic procedures.
- You may qualify for surgery if you have a BMI of 35 or greater without the presence of comorbidities or a BMI of 30–35 with comorbidities.[34]
- Lifestyle changes are crucial before and after bariatric surgery.

For journal prompts related to this chapter and resources on where to start if you are considering surgery to head to www.thesleeveddietitian.com/ea

[34] ASMBS, "Who Is a Candidate?"

Chapter 3
Weight Stigma and Bias

stig·ma

/ˈstigmə/

noun

1. a mark of disgrace associated with a particular circumstance, quality, or person

"The stigma that people with obesity are lazy creates a barrier to beneficial healthcare."

The Glaring Issue of Weight Stigma & Bias

I wish I could tell you that weight stigma was dead. I wish that judging people based on their weight was something we let the early 2000s keep. But I mustn't tell lies. Anyone who has lived in a larger body can tell you firsthand that weight stigma is alive and well. And while I think our society as a whole has become more accepting of people living in larger bodies, there is still a lot of work to do.

By definition, weight stigma refers to the "discriminatory acts and ideologies targeted toward individuals because of their weight and size."[35] Weight stigma is a result of weight bias.[36] Weight bias refers to the negative ideologies associated with obesity.[37]

Weight stigma and bias come in different forms. These are the preconceived

[35] "Weight Stigma," "What We Do: Our Policy Priorities" section on World Obesity Federation website, accessed July 14, 2023, https://www.worldobesity.org/what-we-do/our-policy-priorities/weight-stigma.
[36] World Obesity Federation, "Weight Stigma."
[37] World Obesity Federation, "Weight Stigma."

notions that one might have about a person based on their weight and body size alone. Some of these stigmas include the ideas that . . .

- Fat people are lazy or have terrible work ethic.
- Fat people don't care about themselves or take pride in themselves.
- Fat people are stupid or unintelligent.
- Fat people lack willpower or determination.
- Fat people are unhealthy.

Just to name a few. Anyone who has spent even five seconds on social media could tell you that these biases exist. Anyone who is not actively trying to lose weight and posts content online in a larger body is usually met with comments like "stop glorifying obesity" or "promoting obesity isn't healthy."

To that I say, *No shit, Sherlock*. As a society, we KNOW that carrying significant extra weight on one's body is often (NOT always) a contributor to other health issues. But that's not the problem here. The problem here is the strangers on the internet who are judging and projecting their own beliefs surrounding obesity onto those who are actually experiencing it.

Weight Stigma I Experienced as a Patient in a Larger Body

As bad as it is to have trolls on Instagram judging people because of their body size, what's even worse is when professionals working in healthcare are the ones perpetuating the stigmas.

Unfortunately, there are still many health practitioners who carry around their own assumptions about people in larger bodies. Some of the biggest ones being that people in larger bodies are incompetent, unintelligent, and "noncompliant."

In actuality, weight has no bearing on one's intellectual abilities or compliance. And most people who are at the point of approaching bariatric surgery are also people who have been on a multitude of diets since childhood. Even before I obtained my dietetics degree, I could rattle off the calories of any given product at any given time—because diet culture, while all-consuming and detrimental as hell—has taught us how to read a label inside and out to look for the most minuscule of details. So to assume that someone, because they are in a bariatric-sized body, must not know their ass from their elbow is, quite frankly, insulting.

When I was about two months shy of starting my pre-op liquid diet, I had an appointment at my bariatric center. I made a comment to the medical assistant about how, after my appointment, I had to rush back to class. The assistant pulled out the plus-size blood pressure cuff and wrapped it around my arm. She asked what I was going to school for, and I proudly said, "I'm finishing up my dietetic internship. I'm going to be a registered dietitian."

The medical assistant paused and looked at me, then she burst out laughing. Not just a chuckle, but a full-blown big belly laugh, as if she had just heard the funniest joke imaginable.

I looked down at the floor, hurt and holding back tears. I felt ashamed.

She then snorted, "Wow, okay," and left the room while I waited for my surgeon to come in.

I held back tears my entire appointment. I was good at it; I always had been. Years of hiding the hurt you feel makes you pretty good at it. But looking back, I realize I should have said something. I should have stood up for myself. I honestly should have reported her. But I didn't.

Was she right? Could a fat dietitian actually help anyone? The girl who needed bariatric surgery thought she was going to help people succeed with their own weight loss? Yeah right.

But I guess the joke's on her.

I wish I could go back and tell myself in that moment that I was enough and I have always been enough—that I was capable of accomplishing every single dream I had. Since that day, I vowed to make it my mission to stand up for this community. To advocate for people going through weight loss surgery and to advocate for people living in larger bodies. I vowed to make sure no one ever felt the way I felt that day, so long as it was on my watch. I vowed to do better and be better for this community. You deserve better. I deserved better. We all deserve better.

Stigma Around Weight Loss Surgery (WLS)

Isn't it funny that people discriminate so openly and unapologetically against people in larger bodies while simultaneously shitting on them once they take the action steps needed to lose weight?

Viral memes, similar to the one above, pretty accurately sum up how much of our society views bariatrics (surgery and medication management) for obesity.

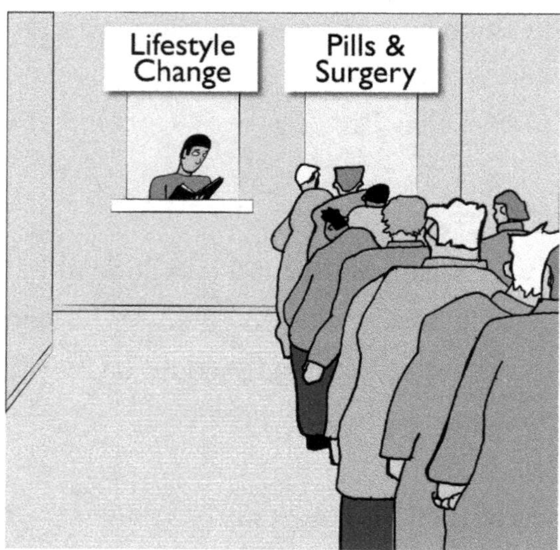

Cartoon graphic showing a long line of people lining up beneath a sign that reads "pills and surgery" as well as an empty line beneath a sign that reads "lifestyle change."

There seems to be this wild assumption that people who choose to treat their obesity through bariatrics are somehow looking for some kind of "quick fix." There's this assumption that people in our society don't want to work for their weight loss, going back to the stigma of being "lazy" or "unmotivated."

The thing that most don't realize is that people who opt for surgery or medication are not trying to find a loophole. They aren't trying to find a work-around for having to eat well, exercise, etc. They simply want to be able to do those things and have them actually yield the results they have been working so hard for with little success.

If lifestyle changes alone worked for treating obesity, no one would feel inclined to seek out other tools and options. Lifestyle changes will ALWAYS be a PART of the equation, but obesity is a complex disease with so many factors; and for many, lifestyle alone simply is not enough.

What's also interesting (and disheartening) is the hate and shame thrown at bariatric patients from other people who struggle with their weight. One of the terms that is pretty frustrating for bariatric patients to hear is the term "natural weight loss."

If you scroll through weight loss pages on social media, you will find many accounts put "Natural weight loss only, no pills or surgery" in their bios. If you are someone who lost a significant amount of weight without the support of medical interventions, that is amazing. I am proud of you, and what you've done is incredible. But the question I ask you is this: why do you feel like it's important to let the world know you DIDN'T need another tool? Where does that pride come from? Why is that piece important?

When bariatric patients see things like that, it makes them feel shame for needing a tool. As if they didn't try hard enough before surgery or medications. As if something is wrong with them. As if they are a failure.

And let me just say this: no one, not one person, opts for surgery before trying to "do it on their own" first. Did you know that, in the US, in order to be approved by insurance for weight loss surgery, you need to show that you've made previous unsuccessful attempts at weight loss first? As much as I hate that surgery is most people's last resort, that's usually the case.

Imagine how many more people would overcome obesity sooner, living longer and healthier lives, if surgery wasn't seen as shameful and wasn't considered a last resort. What if it was an option presented to people sooner? Why does one's weight need to get so out of control before surgery is an option?

Maybe if the world stopped shaming people for asking for help, people would actually get the help they need and deserve sooner.

Weight Stigma I Witnessed Working with Other Healthcare Professionals

Personally experiencing weight stigma is absolutely debilitating. It eats at your self-worth and cuts so very deep. It's devastating. But to watch others experience weight stigma? To watch your colleagues treat their patients with such bias? It's absolutely and utterly enraging.

After I finished up my dietetic internship, I immediately got a job as a clinical dietitian working in long-term care. It certainly wasn't my dream job, but I was grateful nonetheless and needed the experience (and the paycheck). I expected this job to be hard for a lot of reasons. Caring for medically compromised patients, having to stay on top of diligent charting, and being familiar with end-of-life care were some of my biggest concerns. I guess it didn't occur to me that, on top of all of those hard tasks, I would also be dealing with physicians, nurses, and therapists who outwardly displayed a distaste for obese and bariatric patients.

One day, while sitting in on morning rounds, I heard the team discussing whether or not to admit a patient who needed a "bariatric bed." (For those who may not know, a "bariatric bed" doesn't refer to equipment needed for a weight loss surgery patient; it refers to a bed frame that can support a patient of up to 750 lbs.)

When the discussion of this patient came up, the team unanimously groaned.

"Ugh, another one?"

"No way. They're noncompliant and so hard to take care of."

"I'm not taking care of that patient. I have enough on my plate."

I sat there bewildered. Saddened. Enraged.

I learned very quickly that certain practitioners had a strong distaste for severely obese patients. In their minds, all these patients were one and the same: they would be a lot of work, challenging to deal with, and "noncompliant," so why bother?

I encountered this again while on the floor at the nurses' station one day, going through medical charts before seeing my patients. One of the respiratory therapists, who also complained about how challenging it was to work with obese patients, pulled me aside to ask me some of her own personal nutrition questions. (This happens to dietitians a lot, as everyone wants to pick your brain to get your opinion on their new diet or nutrition regimen . . . Well, if you're a dietitian in an already thin body, that is.)

As she was going on about her struggles with her weight and how she wanted to hit her weight loss goals, she said to me, "Maybe I'll just go ahead and get one of those gastric sleeve surgeries everyone's getting, because it would be a lot easier than having to try so hard every day."

"Actually," I responded, "surgery is really challenging. Whether you have surgery or not, you still need to change your habits and put in the work. It's not easy."

Now, mind you, she had absolutely no idea that I'd had surgery, nor did she know me as anything but the "thin" dietitian who worked on her floor.

"Yeah, well, must be nice, as you've clearly never struggled with your weight or had to worry about these things. But yeah, I probably wouldn't get one of those surgeries anyway. I mean, they don't even work! Everyone I've ever known who's actually had surgery just puts all the weight back on."

As she walked away, I once again sat there bewildered. All I could think was, *Did that conversation really just happen?*

If she only knew.

Weight stigma and bias don't only exist for those in large bodies; they exist for those in smaller bodies too. Both are hurtful. Both are not okay.

Bariatric patients usually experience both sides of the coin. For example, maybe you take the leap of faith to have surgery, only to be met with hurtful comments.

"Why don't you just try harder?"

"Have you thought about just exercising and eating less?"

"Oh, you don't need surgery, just do what I did [insert completely unsustainable and unrealistic weight loss method here]."

"Surgery is the easy way out."

Then maybe, despite the judgment and lack of support and being alone and scared, you finally have surgery. You FINALLY start losing weight, shedding the extra pounds, and doing the one thing in your life you always felt like you were supposed to do. And everyone is happy . . . until they're not.

What starts off as, "Wow you look great" can quickly turn into "Are you done losing yet?" or "You're too skinny." This can leave you feeling like, no matter what you do, it will never be enough. No one is ever happy.

How Those Who Love You Sometimes Treat You After Extreme Weight Loss

Weight, whether you are in a larger or smaller body, shouldn't impact your relationships with friends, family, partners, etc. But because our society puts such an emphasis on weight, unfortunately it does.

Our society has created this standard that makes us all feel insecure about our bodies. So sometimes, when you start losing weight, it triggers an insecurity in someone else. Even if it's not intentional, the people around you can get comfortable with you being bigger than they are and internally pride themselves on being smaller than you. Again, it's not usually intentional. It can even be subconscious. This can even occur in friendships and relationships, especially if the foundations of those relationships are a bit rocky to begin with. Dynamics can shift and change when you go through extreme weight loss.

I've encountered, spoken to, and worked with thousands of bariatric patients. I have yet to talk with a person who has not come across this struggle with those around them. I, too, lost friends and family along the way, some of whom I was very close to. One person, in particular, threw in my face, "You've changed, and you're different since you've lost weight."

Yes, yes, I am different. That's kind of the whole point. I'm no longer struggling with my mental or physical health like I was before. I'm no longer sitting on the sidelines of my life. I'm no longer the sidekick friend. I'm the friend who *also* gets attention and compliments when I go out (stay tuned for my discussion on thin privilege), and I'm no longer embarrassed of who I am. I speak my mind and stand up for myself now. And to the people who sling this as an insult, my rebuttal is this: "Yes, I've changed, but why are YOU bothered by that?"

When people react like this, they are usually projecting something deep down that they may not even be aware of. And I'm not even angry or resentful toward those people; they are hurting from the aftermath of weight stigma and bias too. None of us seem to be able to escape it. Weight stigma and bias have a hold on all of us.

Thin or "Skinny" Privilege

Thin privilege is generally defined as "a set of social advantages that thin people have, as a result of prejudice against people who are heavier or less lean."[38] This all circles back to weight bias and weight stigma.

I never gave thin privilege much thought until I was in a smaller body and, for the first time, recognized this new foreign universe I was apparently living in. It's actually wild, because people are genuinely nicer to me now that I'm living in a smaller body.

Aside from the fact that cisgender, heterosexual men treat me WILDLY differently now that I'm in a thinner body, people in general are much kinder to me in day-to-day life.

I'm talking about the random lady at the grocery store who looks me in the eyes and smiles at me. Or the cashier behind the counter at Dunkin' who goes out of his way to make small talk and give me a free coffee. Or the random person who holds the door open for me and acknowledges my presence.

People notice me now. People actually acknowledge me and want to talk to me. People compliment me on my hair, makeup, clothes, etc. People chit-chat with me in line at the store or do small favors for no good reason.

Some of you might be thinking "Well, yeah, Jamie, that's just human decency.

---

[38] "What is Thin Privilege?," "Learn: Health at Every Size" section on Within Health website, last updated October 27, 2022, https://withinhealth.com/learn/articles/what-is-thin-privilege#resources.

That's nothing special."

Oh, but it is.

It IS special when you never experienced this kind of human decency UNTIL you were no longer in a large body. And THAT is thin privilege. I went the first 24 years of my life living in a morbidly obese body. I can promise you, random acts of kindness from strangers were few and far between. I felt unnoticed. And when I was noticed, I felt judged.

There's a reason I've had to learn to walk without looking down at my feet. Out of habit, I still do it. It's easier to keep your head down, stay out of people's way, and avoid eye contact when you're so used to being met with judgmental gazes.

When I talk about thin privilege, I'm usually met with the comment, "Well, you're also more comfortable in your own skin and you're more confident, so the energy you are projecting now is reciprocated." Well, yeah, that might be partially true and play a role as well. But I genuinely feel like people are kinder to me, more likely to look me in the eyes, and more likely to let me have my way or get away with things because I'm in a body society views as acceptable.

Health at Every Size, Body Positivity, and Intuitive Eating: Are They Really Helping to Combat the Stigmas and Improve Health Outcomes for Those in Larger Bodies?

I would be doing you an extreme disservice if I talked about weight stigma and bias without shining light on the conversations surrounding Health at Every Size (HAES), the Body Positivity Movement (BoPo), and intuitive eating (IE). Buckle up for this one, because what I have to say might not be what you expect.

I don't think that the BoPo Movement, HAES, or IE are singularly problematic. In fact, I use quite a few of these principles and beliefs in my own education and framework. There is evidence to support HAES and IE, and as a dietitian, it's my job to use evidence-based nutrition guidance and practices. Plus, I think all of these movements encourage people to show themselves love and care, no matter their weight or their size, by honoring and celebrating their bodies and being in tune with themselves.

I think the principles of these movements—like rejecting toxic diet culture, making peace with food, getting out of the "good-versus-bad" food mentality, listening to and respecting your body, and coping with emotions—are critical, which is why I speak about these things regularly to the weight loss surgery community. The problem lies not in the origins of these principles, but in the way they have been translated into the media and healthcare.

Here's a quick breakdown of what these movements are all about.

HAES: According to The Association for Size Diversity and Health, HAES is "a holistic definition of health, which cannot be characterized as the absence of physical or mental illness, limitation, or disease. Rather, health exists on a continuum that varies with time and circumstance for each individual."[39]

BoPo: The Body Positivity Movement is a movement to accept bodies of all sizes and types, rather than just those that conform to societal ideals of beauty. It emphasizes self-acceptance, inner worth, and appreciation for a body's abilities.[40]

IE: Intuitive Eating is an evidence-based, mind-body health approach created by registered dietitians Evelyn Tribole and Elyse Resch in 1995 that is composed of ten principles, including rejecting the diet mentality, honoring your hunger, making peace with food, feeling your fullness, respecting your body,

---

[39] "About Health at Every Size (HAES)," "Health at Every Size Principles" on Association for Size Diversity and Health website, accessed July 14, 2023, https://asdah.org/health-at-every-size-haes-approach/.
[40] "Body Positivity," "Get Help: Basics" section on PsychologyToday.com, accessed July 14, 2023, https://www.psychologytoday.com/us/basics/body-positivity.

and more.[41]

Let's start with HAES and IE, as they have a lot of crossover. Even though HAES and IE aim to advance and improve healthcare outcomes, and in certain scenarios accomplish this, for those struggling with morbid obesity and its comorbidities, I actually believe these principles and messages can be harmful and limiting.

What started off as anti-diet approaches and body positivity have unfortunately turned into an anti-weight-loss movement. IE framework is clear about the fact that IE should never be used with intentional weight loss, and HAES conforms to the idea that weight should not be the main health factor emphasized when discussing health outcomes.[42] Everyone deserves equal access to nondiscriminatory care, but the irony is this actually becomes discriminatory when those who wish to receive treatment for their obesity and comorbidities are ignored or invalidated.

For example, I've worked with multiple people who explicitly told me that they had to find a new dietitian because their previous one labeled themselves as an "anti-diet and HAES" dietitian and, therefore, refused to support them in their pursuits of weight loss and weight loss surgery. I have heard the same thing in regards to "anti-diet and HAES" therapists, who dismissed people from their services because they didn't approve of their decision for surgery.

Bariatrics is a specialty, both in dietetics and therapy. I can completely respect a clinician who recognizes and acknowledges that they don't have the knowledge or skill set to support someone through weight loss surgery. But in that event, the ethical thing to do would be to share that honestly with your patient, and then refer them to someone who is better suited to support them.

---

[41] Evelyn Tribole, "What Is Intuitive Eating?," evelyntribole.com "Blog" page, published September 12, 2018, https://www.evelyntribole.com/what-is-intuitive-eating/.

[42] Evelyn Tribole, "No Health Professional Can Rightly Say You Will Lose Weight with Intuitive Eating, Including Me!," evelyntribole.com "Blog" page, published April 5, 2019, https://www.evelyntribole.com/no-health-professional-can-rightly-say-you-will-lose-weight-with-intuitive-eating-including-me/,

Plus, in my opinion, there is really no such thing as an anti-diet or anti-weight-loss dietitian. We are all simply registered dietitians, with the same schooling, same credentialing parameters, and same code of ethics. The Code of Ethics for the Nutrition and Dietetics Profession includes four main principles: non-maleficence (competence and professional development in practice), autonomy (integrity in personal and organizational behaviors and practices), beneficence (professionalism), and justice (social responsibility for local, regional, national, and global nutrition and well-being).[43] I'm not saying dietitians who dismiss their patients because they don't agree with their choice to lose weight or have weight loss surgery are unethical, but it doesn't *exactly* sound like they're upholding the above principles either.

ALL dietitians should be rejecting fad diets and toxic diet-culture gimmicks, because they are NOT evidence based. ALL dietitians should be supporting their morbidly obese clients in their pursuits for weight loss if it's desired in ways that ARE evidence based.

Someone struggling with obesity and comorbidities needs more than a "gentle nutrition" approach, which is advocated by both IE and HAES. Medical nutrition therapy (MNT) is what registered dietitians are specialized to do when it comes to clinically improving people's health, and this *always* requires a prescriptive diet. People with diabetes are supported with carb-controlled diets. People with heart disease are supported with low-sodium and/or low-fat diets. People with gout are supported with a low-purine diet. People who are clinically underweight are given an increase of calories in their diet. So why is it that some clinicians are rejecting prescribed, evidence-based diets and interventions for their overweight patients? Could it maybe just be . . . weight stigma, perhaps?

In addition to gentle nutrition, another IE and HAES principle that fails to be

[43] Academy of Nutrition and Dietetics, "Code of Ethics for the Nutrition and Dietetics Profession," published 2018, https://www.eatrightpro.org/-/media/files/eatrightpro/practice/code-of-ethics/codeofethicshandout.pdf.

inclusive is the idea that movement should be joyful. As someone who used to be morbidly obese, and as someone who works with bariatric patients, I find this concept ignorant. When your weight is so high that your body can no longer carry you to walk or be mobile, the words "joyful" and "movement" do not go in the same sentence.

Last year, I worked with a client who was five feet tall and about four hundred pounds at her heaviest. She was in pain all the time. Even laying in bed was painful for her. She simply wanted to be able to walk up the stairs to do her laundry without pain. Encouraging her to find "joyful movement" would have been completely dismissive of her struggles and concerns.

It's also important to understand that people with obesity usually have increased hunger and decreased satiety. When someone has increased ghrelin (the hunger hormone) signaling and decreased leptin (the satiety hormone) secretion, it can be difficult and downright ineffective for them to follow the IE principles of "honoring your hunger" and "discovering the satisfaction factor."

It's clear to me that the founders of HAES and IE have a poor understanding of the physiology and complexities surrounding obesity. These principles and beliefs only work some of the time, with some people. Once again, it feels like those in larger bodies are being discriminated against by something that claims to protect them.

Unfortunately, there are similar issues with unintentional discrimination and ironies in the Body Positivity Movement. Just like with HAES and IE, a lot of BoPo and fat-liberation messaging ends up being misconstrued to support ananti-weight-loss narrative. People in the bariatric community often feel shunned by those who subscribe to the BoPo movement, made to feel guilty for choosing to lose weight.

I think it's only fair to first give a bit of context to the BoPo movement. BoPo was not originally intended for White women, and the history behind it is much more complicated than it's been made out to be. The point of the BoPo movement isn't necessarily for everyone to simply just "love" their bodies or feel positively about them, but rather, to take a stance against social norms and pressures of what society says beauty "should" be by bringing adequate representation to people of color, people of different ethnicities, people from LGBTQIA+ communities, older adults, and those with disabilities.[44]

But rather than bringing adequate representation and diversity to society's ideal body standards, what has unfortunately happened is that many thin, fit, White, and conventionally attractive people, specifically cisgender White women, have taken its message to simply be "love yourself despite your 'imperfections.'" They've taken something that wasn't meant for them to be used to further validate their own beauty standards.

I share all of this with you because I think it's important to acknowledge the ways in which the intentions of the BoPo movement have been altered and misconstrued. I don't think it would be fair of me to make commentary on the BoPo movement, and the harm I think it can do to the bariatric community or people seeking treatment for obesity, without giving adequate context and acknowledging the harm that's also been done to those it was meant for.

As someone who used to live in a large body, I really honored and valued the BoPo movement. It inspired me in a lot of ways, even if I struggled to fully accept myself and my body at the time. At the very least, it felt like a safe place where I belonged.

Until it wasn't.

While my experience isn't everyone's, personally, I have been at the receiving end of some of the cruelest comments and accusations from BoPo influencers and advocates. I've been told I'm "unethical" for supporting weight loss sur-

[44] Mary West, "What to Know about the Body Positivity Movement," Medical News Today website, published April 29, 2022, https://www.medicalnewstoday.com/articles/body-positivity#goals.

gery. I've been told "it's barbaric" and a slew of similar accusations. I've even been accused of causing harm to others by sharing about and advocating for surgery.

I suppose that circles back to one's definition of harm. Weight loss, in and of itself, is not inherently harmful. But unfortunately, the opposite belief seems to be the general consensus within the BoPo community. This anti-weight-loss narrative is one of the reasons SO many people refuse to seek out treatment or support. They feel as though it is somehow "wrong" to want or need to lose weight.

And it comes back, once again, to there being all too much emphasis on someone's appearance, rather than their mental, physical, or emotional state. I'm not assuming everyone who is at a higher body weight is unhealthy in any or all of these categories. But for those who are, and who desire to seek treatment through means of intentional weight loss, it can really keep them stuck from seeking help or support.

At my heaviest weight, I was technically healthy "on paper." At the time, I didn't have any other comorbidities or ailments (aside from my PCOS, anyway). But the way I felt emotionally and mentally was anything but healthy. I am a firm believer that if your weight is impacting your social, occupational, spiritual, emotional, or mental health, then you are not healthy.

It is not always possible to achieve health at every size, for everyone, despite how nice that sounds. For some sure, but not all. It's not always possible to eat intuitively, despite how nice it sounds. And it's not always in your best interest to avoid losing weight for the sake of fighting social norms, no matter how badly you might want to.

And this may ruffle some feathers, but you are also *allowed* to want to lose weight for more than just health reasons. If you enjoy the way you feel, the way you look in the mirror, and the way you fit into clothes and the world around you living in a smaller body, you are allowed to. You're allowed to like how you feel in your smaller body. It's not a personal attack towards anyone else or any other body types if you personally choose this path for yourself. It does not mean you are "fatphobic," and it does not make you a hypocrite. You're also allowed to like who you are and how you feel in a larger body. And you are allowed to feel good and healthy in a larger body without being accused of terrible things that coincide with weight stigma and bias.

If you simply just don't want to live in a larger body, that is a valid enough reason to choose to lose weight or have surgery. You have the autonomy to choose without conforming to the pressures and biases around you.

Bite-Sized Recap

- Weight stigma refers to the "discriminatory acts and ideologies targeted toward individuals because of their weight and size." Weight stigma is a result of weight bias.[45]
- Weight bias refers to the negative ideologies associated with obesity.[46]
- Weight stigma happens often, even from those working in the medical field.
- There is a stigma around weight loss surgery. Many label it as an "easy fix" or the "easy way out."
- Some of the ideologies and messages surrounding Healthy at Any Size (HAES), Body Positivity (BoPo), and intuitive eating (IE) can be harmful to the bariatric community or anyone seeking treatment for obesity.
- You have full autonomy over your body and your choice to change it or not. It is okay to want to receive treatment for obesity. It is okay to desire weight loss, and it doesn't make you a bad person, nor does it make you fatphobic.

For journal prompts and resources related to this chapter be sure to head to www.thesleeveddietitian.com/easy.

[45] World Obesity Federation, "Weight Stigma."
[46] World Obesity Federation, "Weight Stigma."

Chapter 4
Anti-Obesity Medications: The History and How They Work

med·i·ca·tion

/medəkāSH(ə)n/

noun

plural noun: medications

1. a substance used for medical treatment, especially a medicine or drug

"certain medications can treat and manage chronic diseases"

My Experience with Weight Loss Medications

Despite my lifelong battle with weight, I never put much thought and consideration into weight loss medications. When I was 14, I was put on a medication called metformin for insulin resistance and PCOS treatment. I had some pretty nasty side effects from that one, including nausea, vomiting, and hot and cold sweats. I also did not lose any weight on it, so after I transitioned off that medication, the thought of pursuing another one never crossed my mind. It wasn't until many years after I had my weight loss surgery that I started to learn what these medications were and who should use them.

After maintaining my 112 pound weight loss for nearly two years, in 2020, I started to struggle with my weight again out of nowhere. Now, I know what you're probably thinking, *Duh, Jamie, that was the year we all endured a global pandemic. Everyone gained weight.* The thing is, though, I don't think that was it. I had quit my full-time clinical job to work from home, which was actually far less stressful and allowed me more control in prepping my meals, and I was actually spending a lot more time walking and working out, because I had the time.

The only other thing that changed was that, in August, I had my IUD removed after having it since before my vertical sleeve gastrectomy. Until this point, I had maintained my weight beautifully, and I felt really confident in my habits and routine. I do suspect that this change in birth control, coinciding with hormonal shifts, played a role in my weight and my body. Because by October, I had jumped up nearly 15 lbs. It felt like this had happened overnight.

I'm not going to lie, I panicked. I knew something deeper was going on, because it just didn't make sense. So I called my surgeon and scheduled an appointment with her. I sat down with both her and one of the dietitians (because, yes, sometimes even dietitians need dietitians), and they both said, "You're doing great; you don't need to change anything." But while they were still happy with my overall progress, I was not. I was alarmed and concerned, and I felt like my fear was brushed off. My surgeon told me that she couldn't help me unless I wanted to have a bariatric surgery revision, which I didn't. There were no other options. She didn't support weight loss medications, so she would not prescribe me one.

The next few years, I really felt like I was "white-knuckling it" just to keep the scale from moving up. I couldn't believe I had to work so hard just to *not* gain weight. For the first time since my surgery, I felt like I was back to where I was before, constantly fighting my body and the scale. Worse than fighting those numbers was the mental struggle of it all. I felt like I was failing. I felt like a hypocrite. Here I was, helping other women on their bariatric journeys while struggling so hard myself. To top it off, my PCOS symptoms that I had once felt so free from were also back with a vengeance. Acne, irregular periods, and weight struggles were a reality for me once again.

In June 2022, I traveled to Dallas for the ASMBS Conference. I sat in on a panel with various surgeons, dietitians, and obesity-certified physicians and nurse practitioners talking about how medication management can significantly help bariatric surgery patients to maintain their weight long term.

One of the speakers said, "How do we support our patients when they regain? Not *if* they regain, *when*. Because no one will stay at their lowest."

Her words struck me hard. But they also brought me an immense amount of comfort. Statistically, most bariatric patients are anticipated to lose as much as 60–77% of their excess weight in the first two years, and on average, maintain 50% of that loss after five years.[47] Which means, statistically speaking, most patients will gain back 10–17% of their weight.

But even though I did fall into this range and was deemed a "bariatric success" by these standards, I was nearing the higher end of that 17%, and I simply was not okay with that. Luckily, I met another dietitian at the conference, who'd also had surgery, just like me. She shared that she was on a GLP-1 medication called Saxenda, one of the medications discussed during the panel, which she started after experiencing some regain. When she started the medication, she was able to lose the regain and maintain it with ease. She said it was the best thing she ever did on her journey.

She inspired me and made me realize that it was, once again, okay to ask for help. I suddenly felt the way I had felt when I was considering surgery: scared, nervous. But I also knew I deserved the help that was available just as much as anyone else. I did not want to sit and wait until it got "bad enough." I didn't want to be a sitting duck, fighting my body tooth and nail, only to wake up one day back to where I started. I was not going to let that happen.

I started doing my own research. I ended up reaching out to Dr. Spencer Nadolsky, an obesity and lipid specialist, and in August 2022, after two full years of struggling, I was prescribed a medication called Mounjaro.

This medication has changed my life. So much so, I honestly wonder how my journey might have played out differently had this been an option for me before I had surgery. I want to be very clear: I do *not* regret my weight loss sur-

---

[47] ASMBS, "U.S. Obesity Rate Higher Than Ever."

gery. It was the best decision I have ever made. But getting on this medication has been a very close second.

Since August 2022, not only am I down 45 pounds. (surpassing my previous lowest adult weight), but I can truthfully say I have never felt this good mentally in my entire life. It's not because of the weight loss either. Since being on this medication, my brain is different. All the obsessive food thoughts I've had to fight day in and day out my whole life are gone. My worry about my weight even seems to be gone. For the first time, it's quiet. I don't think about what I will or will not eat all day. I don't think about my food choices in an obsessive or self-deprecating way. I don't feel like I need to restrict myself. I've had zero urge to binge. It's the wildest thing.

I only think about food when I'm genuinely hungry. And when I'm hungry, I eat, and I'm able to stop as soon as I'm full without pushing or overdoing it. If this is what people who don't have food or weight issues feel like, no wonder they don't have weight issues.

The Evolution of Weight Loss Medications

Anti-obesity medications, or AOMs, are the second branch of medicine within the field of bariatrics. AOMs can be incredibly life-changing for many people, but they haven't always gotten the best reputation. The biggest reason for this is that, until recently, the majority of weight loss medications on the market were proven to be rather *ineffective*, with many serious side effects.

It's only been within the last ten years that adequate and effective AOMs have come about. In the meantime, over the last few decades, over-the-counter stimulants such as Hydroxycut and other "fat burners" (which are supplements, not medications) have become a popular alternative to AOMs. This is because, as always, the diet industry took them and ran, labeling them as "diet pills."

Diet pills, like those over-the-counter stimulants, have gotten a really bad reputation for ineffective, short-term results, and side effects. The FDA has repeatedly warned consumers about the risks of weight loss supplements, as these supplements are NOT regulated by the FDA, do not undergo the same testing or clinical studies that medications undergo today, and often include anorectics or appetite suppressants—which can include derivatives of amphetamines.[48]

I think even the term "diet pill" has a very different connotation attached to it than the term "anti-obesity medication." AOMs are coined as a "quick fix," and this misrepresentation of what they truly are has contributed to the stigma and the controversies surrounding them.

The complex history of AOMs dates as far back as the late 1890s, when the first medication to treat hypothyroidism, with a significant impact on weight, emerged.[49] As we moved through the decades, more AOMs came to the market, including Obetrol (a combination of amphetamine salts that included methamphetamine) which was the start of the "Rainbow Pill Period," referring to a type of polypharmacy where amphetamines were being prescribed with additional medications to counteract the stimulant effect.[50]

There were many other medications to come, many of which have been pulled from the market entirely due to their ineffectiveness, side effects, and risk factors.[51] One that's stuck around is phentermine. In the 1990s, phentermine began being combined with other weight loss drugs, like fenfluramine and dexfenfluramine, to make what was referred to as "fen-phen" pills. Unfortunately, significant health problems like heart issues were reported, and the

---

[48] Pieter A. Cohen et al., "The Return of Rainbow Diet Pills," *American Journal of Public Health* 102, no. 9 (September 2012): 1676–1686, https://www.ncbi.nlm.nih.gov/pmc/articles/PMC3482033/,

[49] George A. Bray and Jonathan Purnell, "An Historical Review of Steps and Missteps in the Discovery of Anti-Obesity Drugs," in K. R. Feingold et al., eds., *Endotext* [Internet], South Dartmouth, MA: MDtext.com, 2000–, last updated July 10, 2022, available at https://www.ncbi.nlm.nih.gov/books/NBK581942/.

[50] T. D. Müller et al., "Anti-Obesity Therapy: From Rainbow Pills to Polyagonists," *Pharmacological Reviews* 70, no. 4 (October 2018): 712–746, https://pharmrev.aspetjournals.org/content/70/4/712.

[51] Katey Davidson and Gavin Van De Walle, "Does Phentermine Work for Weight Loss? A Diet Pill Reviewed," "Nutrition" section on Healthline.com, last updated February 3, 2023, https://www.healthline.com/nutrition/phentermine-weight-loss#what-it-is.

FDA pulled fenfluramine and dexfenfluramine from the market.[52] Today, the singular form phentermine, known as Suprenza, can still be used on its own for up to 12 weeks. Alternatively, Qsymia, a drug combining phentermine with topiramate, can be taken long term.

Few drugs prior to phentermine made headway, or even made it to approval, due to severe side effects such as addiction, neuropathy, and total ineffectiveness.[53] Thankfully, Western medicine has evolved drastically since then, in all regards, and there have been plenty of scientific advances with AOMs.

In their 2012 article, "Anti-obesity Drugs: Past, Present and Future," researchers R. John Rodgers, Matthias H. Tschöp, and John P. H. Wilding said:

> The ideal anti-obesity drug would produce sustained weight loss with minimal side effects. The mechanisms that regulate energy balance have substantial built-in redundancy, overlap considerably with other physiological functions, and are influenced by social, hedonic and psychological factors that limit the effectiveness of pharmacological interventions . . . It is therefore unsurprising that anti-obesity drug discovery programmes have been littered with false starts, failures in clinical development, and withdrawals due to adverse effects that were not fully appreciated at the time of launch. Drugs that target pathways in metabolic tissues, such as adipocytes, liver and skeletal muscle, have shown potential in preclinical studies but none has yet reached clinical development.[54]

These researchers were touching on something that later became critical in the world of obesity and weight management. If you are even slightly familiar with this world, then you have definitely heard about the latest craze: the "weight loss injections" taking the country by storm. These "weight loss injections" are

[52] Müller et al., "Anti-Obesity Therapy."
[53] Bray and Purnell, "Steps and Missteps in the Discovery of Anti-Obesity Drugs."
[54] R. John Rodgers et al., "Anti-Obesity Drugs: Past, Present, and Future," *Disease Models and Mechanisms* 5, no. 5 (September 2012): 621–626, https://www.ncbi.nlm.nih.gov/pmc/articles/PMC3424459/.

actually GLP-1 medications, a classification of weight loss medication that was first approved for DM2 management in 2005 by the FDA.[55]

The discovery, characteristics, and clinical development of GLP-1 dates back more than 30 years.[56] GLP-1 is a peptide hormone that has a pretty profound effect on enhancing insulin secretion and an incredible effect on decreasing gastric motility, keeping people fuller longer and increasing satiety.

Researchers R. John Rodgers, Matthias H. Tschöp, and John P. H. Wilding actually predicted the effectiveness of GLP-1 medications in that very same article from 2012:

> Recent improvements in the understanding of peptidergic signaling of hunger and satiety from the gastrointestinal tract mediated by ghrelin, cholecystokinin (CCK), peptide YY (PYY) and glucagon-like peptide-1 (GLP-1), and of homeostatic mechanisms related to leptin and its upstream pathways in the hypothalamus, have opened up new possibilities. Although some have now reached clinical development, it is uncertain whether they will meet the strict regulatory hurdles required for licensing of an anti-obesity drug. However, GLP-1 receptor agonists have already succeeded in diabetes treatment and, owing to their attractive body-weight-lowering effects in humans, will perhaps also pave the way for other anti-obesity agents.[57]

If that's a whole lot of science jargon for you, more simply put, what they were saying was that GLP-1 was already known to keep people fuller and more satisfied and help with overall weight reduction. They were speculating that if GLP-1 medications could withstand the rigorous testing and hurdles it would take to become FDA approved for obesity management, these medications would likely have a substantial impact on AOMs as we know them.

---

[55] R. John Rodgers et al.,, "Anti-Obesity Drugs."
[56] R. John Rodgers et al.,, "Anti-Obesity Drugs."
[57] R. John Rodgers et al.,, "Anti-Obesity Drugs."

And boy were they right! Because now here we are, with what truly appears to be the most "perfect" weight loss medication for those who struggle with obesity. However, all good things seem to come at a cost (both literally and figuratively). And although we finally have the most promising AOM to date, and with more to come, it has received a lot of criticism. This is largely because many people in Hollywood and in affluent communities are taking these medications when obesity and diabetes are NOT indicated to achieve an unnatural, dangerous level of thinness. In other words, they are being abused and portrayed as a harmful "trend."

Between this and the complicated history of AOMs, I can completely understand where the criticism is coming from. I don't even blame the people who are skeptical. You SHOULD be skeptical. But the problem is, although the research is there, all people are hearing and seeing is what the tabloids are portraying. And while these medications may appear to be "trendy" because of their Hollywood popularity, the truth is that they are truly groundbreaking in the field of bariatrics.

GLP-1 Medications and How They Work

Looking at that data, it really is quite remarkable how effective the GLP-1 medications are. While the exact mechanisms are still being researched and understood, it appears that GLP-1 plays a role in regulating glucose metabolism and food intake, as well as impacting the major neural pathways in the brain that influence eating behaviors.[58]

The three most common GLP-1 medications being used for weight loss at this time are Ozempic, Wegovy, and Mounjaro, all of which are subcutaneous (under the skin), injectable medications. Ozempic and Mounjaro are currently FDA approved for the treatment of type 2 diabetes, and Wegovy is specifically

[58] Charlotte C. Ronveaux et al., "Glucagon-Like Peptide 1 Interacts with Ghrelin and Leptin to Regulate Glucose Metabolism and Food Intake through Vagal Afferent Neuron Signaling," *Journal of Nutrition* 145, no. 4 (February 2015): 672–680, https://www.ncbi.nlm.nih.gov/pmc/articles/PMC4381768/.

FDA approved to treat obesity. Oftentimes, Ozempic and Mounaro are prescribed off-label for obesity treatment due to the remarkable effect they have on weight management.[59]

Ozempic and Wegovy both use semaglutide as their main ingredient. Wegovy is FDA approved for weight loss, while Ozempic currently is not. Semaglutide is a GLP-1 receptor agonist, so when someone takes a semaglutide injection, the semaglutide binds to the GLP-1 receptors and stimulates the pancreas to release insulin. The reason it helps with weight loss is because it slows down gastric emptying, which is the rate at which food moves through the digestive system.[60] This process helps a person feel fuller longer, which reduces overall food intake and consumption, hence, resulting in weight loss.

Mounjaro's main ingredient is Tirezpatide, a dual-acting GIP (glucose-dependent insulinotropic polypeptide) and GLP-1 receptor agonist. So in addition to everything that semaglutide does, Tirezpatide also lowers fasting and postprandial glucose concentration, further decreasing food intake, increasing satiety, and aiding people in weight loss.[61] While Mounjaro is not yet FDA approved for weight loss, it is currently undergoing fast-track designation for the treatment of adults with obesity.[62]

In the Phase 3 SURMOUNT-1 study published in 2022, weight loss results from the use of Mounjaro were compared to a placebo group.[63] This 72-week study followed the two groups of patients, both of which did not have type 2 diabetes and underwent intense lifestyle changes. It found that 50–57% of patients achieved a weight loss of 20% or more, compared to just a 3% loss in

---

[59] Leigh Ann Anderson, "How Do Mounjaro, Wegovy & Ozempic Compare for Weight Loss?," "Medical Answers" section of Drugs.com website, https://www.drugs.com/medical-answers/mounjaro-wegovy-ozempic-compare-weight-loss-3570898/.

[60] Anderson, "Mounjaro, Wegovy & Ozempic."

[61] Anderson, "Mounjaro, Wegovy & Ozempic."

[62] Anderson, "Mounjaro, Wegovy & Ozempic."

[63] You can learn more about the ongoing SURMOUNT-1 Clinical Trials here: https://classic.clinicaltrials.gov/ct2/show/NCT04184622&sa=D&source=docs&ust=1689299623524195&usg=AOvVaw3EcoG21QH6KDtfT7C3Oe0T.

the placebo group.[64] That is a HUGE difference. This amount of weight loss approaches numbers typically only seen as a result of bariatric surgery.

Other GLP-1 medications are being studied, including CagriSema, a dual-acting GLP-1/GIP/glucagon agonist. CagriSema seems to emulate **amylin**, which is a hormone secreted from the pancreas to increase satiety. It also contains **retatrutide**, which not only helps with satiety and fullness, but also helps people burn more calories.[65]

Medication Management in Conjunction with Bariatric Surgery

When it comes to treating obesity with bariatrics (surgical treatment and medications), it's not always one or the other. Sometimes, it's both. The ASMBS is in favor of AOMs in both the pre-operative and postoperative bariatric setting when indicated and appropriate. It's been shown that AOMs can be beneficial both in helping with weight reduction prior to getting surgical approval, often making surgery safer for patients, as well as with weight maintenance or weight regain after surgery.

In 2021, the ASMBS Clinical Issues Committee performed a literature review assessing AOMs in surgical patients. They stated, "AOMs should be used in conjunction with intensive lifestyle changes that incorporate caloric modification, physical activity, and healthy nutrition."[66] So just to be crystal clear, no one—and I mean NO ONE—is suggesting that someone should have surgery, go on medication, or use both treatment options without implementing healthy habits and lifestyle changes too. Lifestyle changes will always play a HUGE role in weight management.

---

[64] Anderson, "Mounjaro, Wegovy & Ozempic."

[65] Spencer Nadolsky and Amelia Harnish, "The Next Generation of Weight-Loss Drugs Will Be Even More Powerful than Ozempic," *Women's Health Magazine* website, published January 31, 2023, https://www.womenshealthmag.com/weight-loss/a42623753/weight-loss-drugs-future-ozempic-wegovy-mounjaro/.

[66] R. Wesley Vosburg et al., "Literature Review on Antiobesity Medication Use for Metabolic and Bariatric Surgery Patients from the American Society for Metabolic and Bariatric Surgery Clinical Issues Committee," *Surgery for Obesity and Related Diseases* 18 (2022), 1109–1119, https://asmbs.org/app/uploads/2022/09/PIIS1550728922005755.pdf.

In addition to the data and studies that show GLP-1 medications may be incredibly effective for pre- and post-surgical bariatric patients, I think we need to take into account the anecdotal experiences and firsthand accounts of surgical patients on these medications.

I've had really meaningful conversations with WLS patients who have also been on GLP-1 medications. The experiences they've shared with me have been overwhelmingly positive and beautiful.

A previous client of mine (who, let me just say, is a badass) came to me at two years post-op VSG, because she was struggling with old habits creeping in—obsessive food thoughts and uncontrollable cravings. We worked together for over six months, tackling her mindset and working on meal planning and nutrition habits. She killed it. She went on to join CrossFit, compete, and really truly take control over her physical and mental health. But despite all her efforts and her constant dedication, she still felt like she was white-knuckling it day in and day out, fighting SO hard just to maintain her weight. So recently, in conjunction with her surgery and all the work she continues to put in, her physician also prescribed her Mounjaro. Knowing I'm on Mounjaro too, and that I've supported her through every struggle, she trusted me enough to reach out.

Through tears, she said, "Jamie, is this how people who don't struggle with their weight feel? Is this what it feels like to be normal? I'm so emotional, because I didn't know it was possible to feel this way. I can't believe I've gone my whole life NOT feeling this way." And to be honest, I cried with her.

This seems to be the universal consensus—that if THIS is how people who don't struggle with their weight feel like, no wonder they don't struggle. When all you've known is insatiable hunger and cravings, deprivation just to lose a few pounds, and constant and obsessive food thoughts and cravings, the quiet and stillness that comes with these medications is euphoric.

Maybe that sounds dramatic to the average person, but you don't know what you don't know. And when you don't know it's possible to NOT obsess about food, the freedom that these medications create is genuinely life-changing.

In a recent survey I sent out to WLS patients on GLP-1 medications, I asked them to describe the feeling of being on the GLP-1 medication in one sentence. Here are just a few of the responses I got:

- "It's renewed my hope!"
- "The silence in my head is amazing."
- "My stomach and my brain are no longer at war with each other."
- "It's taken most of the emotional noise out of my eating and food choices. It's so helpful."
- "I feel great! It's helped me get back on track and stop binge-eating episodes, which I never was able to do before."
- "It's allowed me to break through the food noise and spend time working on fixing my habits."
- "It cleared the chatter in my head around food, and I have way less cravings!"
- "It's brought quiet and peace to my mind that I've never experienced; it feels so freeing!"
- "It's allowed me to feel full for the first time ever in my life! I've never felt this way, even after VSG. It has given me hope and the ability to control my portions without white-knuckling it."
- "It's brought me freedom from the mental load of obsessing about food all the time."
- "It has assisted me to choose what fuels my body versus just being impulsive."
- "It's helped give me my life back and to not feel held down by my PCOS."
- "It has made me feel like I'm in control of my body and metabolic systems again."
- "It's allowed me to feel like a 'normal' person and not focus on all the

food noise."

In this survey, I also invited people to share any negative experiences they had on these medications. So far, I have yet to have someone provide a firsthand account of a negative experience or reason they wished they weren't on them. Unanimously, all the people I've spoken to have expressed immense gratitude for being able to be on these medications.

Now, this isn't scientific data, and this isn't "evidence." But I think hearing from WLS patients, firsthand, about how freeing it's been for them is really telling and has got to be worth something.

Being on Mounjaro has changed MY life in ways I never thought possible and never would have imagined. It's brought mental freedom and clarity that even my VSG didn't bring. But for me, personally, I do truly feel like I needed both tools—the surgery and the medication. Having the physical restrictions to manage portions in conjunction with the mental clarity and decrease in appetite and cravings has been the ultimate powerhouse combo. This in addition to all the years of therapy, working on my habits, and working out, has made me feel like everything has FINALLY come together in the most beautiful way possible.

So I don't know that GLP-1s will ever replace bariatric surgery, but I do think they will continue to change the treatment of obesity as we know it. They will likely be utilized first, before surgery, especially for those with a lower BMI. But I think everyone who wants treatment for their obesity and comorbidities needs to put together their own missing puzzle pieces. It's going to look different for everyone.

I don't have all the answers, I don't think anyone does, yet, but I do think we are truly headed in the right direction.

Bite-Sized Recap

- Anti-obesity medications, or AOMs, are the second branch of medicine within the field of bariatrics. AOMs can be incredibly life-changing for many people, but they haven't always gotten the best reputation. Non-FDA-approved "diet pills" and supplements may have negatively contributed to the stigma around AOMs.
- It's only been within the last 10 years that adequate and effective AOMs have come about.
- The complex history of AOMs dates as far back as the late 1890s, when the first medication to treat hypothyroidism emerged with significant impact on weight.[67]
- GLP-1 medications are some of the most effective anti-obesity medications to date.
- When it comes to treating obesity with bariatrics (surgical treatment and medications), it's not always one or the other. Sometimes, it's both. The ASMBS is in favor of AOMs in both the pre-operative and postoperative bariatric setting when indicated and appropriate.
- It's been shown that AOMs can be beneficial in helping with weight reduction prior to getting surgical approval, often making surgery safer for patients, as well as with weight maintenance or weight regain after surgery.

For journal prompts and resources related to this chapter be sure to head to *<u>www.thesleeveddietitian.com/easy</u>*.

[67] Bray and Purnell, "Steps and Missteps in the Discovery of Anti-Obesity Drugs."

Chapter 5
Anti-Obesity Medications: Objections, Stigma, and Other Issues

ob·jec·tion

/*uh*b-jek-sh*uh*n/

noun

1. an expression or feeling of disapproval or opposition; a reason for disagreeing.

"They have raised many objections to the use of medications."

2. the action of challenging or disagreeing with something.

"His view is open to objection."

Objections to GLP-1 Medications and Concerns

Now that we have the history and a few "wins" about AOMs, we're going to dive into the other side. The objections and concerns surrounding GLP-1 medications are valid, and I think you should always be skeptical and ask questions. There are two big questions I continuously hear. The first is this: "What happens when you go off the medication? Won't you just gain the weight back?"

Unfortunately, yes.

When you go off the medication, you will likely regain some, if not all, of the weight you lost while on the medication. The reason these medications are so effective is because they decrease hunger, increase satiety, and target the brain-body connection that makes losing weight so hard for people with obesity. These factors are what enables people to get into a caloric deficit in order to lose weight when they are on these drugs. So naturally, if you come off of them, while you technically still could maintain that calorie deficit, it will be much harder since hunger will be increased, satiety will be decreased, and more intense and even obsessive thoughts surrounding food may come back.

It certainly is possible to come off of the medications, if you want or need to, but I think it's important to understand that most people will gain the weight back if and when they do. While I'm not a physician, and you should always consult with your own doctor or clinician before stopping a medication, if your plan is to come off of the medications, I would suggest that you titrate back down to a lower dosage, just like you titrate up while you are getting on it. This way, the effects aren't so drastic.

However, GLP-1s *are* able to be taken long term. And if they are safe to be taken long term, why wouldn't you want to be on them long term? Obesity is a chronic disease. Even if you get down to a "healthy" or "normal" weight, your battle with obesity will be lifelong. So why wouldn't you treat it chronically as well—especially if it helps you maintain your weight and maintain your health, and allows you the mental and physical freedom to feel better?

If someone has high blood pressure (BP), and they go on a BP medication, their BP will come down. Well, once it goes down, their physician typically won't just take them off. Because what will happen? Their BP will go back up. Same thing with mental health. If someone is put on antianxiety medication, and it effectively manages their anxiety, you wouldn't just abruptly stop taking it. And I'm not suggesting that people never get off of BP or anxiety meds; they do! But there are nuances here, and the same logic should be applied to AOMs.

The second most common question I receive regarding GLP-1 medications is this: "What about the side effects? Aren't the side effects really dangerous and awful?" I can confidently say that one of the reasons these medications have gained such popularity is because they are both effective and safe. The most common side effects reported are nausea, constipation, and/or diarrhea.

Luckily, these side effects seem to be easily managed with anti-nausea and anti-diarrheal medications, as well as fiber supplements, as needed. Plus, once the medications are titrated up and the patient adjusts to their dosage, these side effects tend to lessen or go away completely with time.

Although unlikely, as with all medications, there are going to be black box warnings for potentially serious side effects, which include pancreatitis (inflammation of the pancreas), hypoglycemia (low blood sugar), impaired kidney function, and gallbladder issues.[68] Having a history of these issues may put you at a higher risk for these side effects, which is why it's so important to discuss all possibilities with your physician.

The main contraindication for using GLP-1 medications is a history (or family history) of medullary thyroid carcinoma (MTC). It's important to clarify that MTC is different from having a history of thyroid cancer. There are four different types of thyroid cancer, with MTC being the rarest, making up just 3–4% of all known thyroid cancers.[69]

I'm not minimizing the seriousness of the side effects listed above. They should be taken VERY seriously if you are someone who is at risk for these issues or has a history of them. But for the majority of people, this isn't the case, which is why I think if you are struggling with obesity, it is worth at least having the conversation with your providers to see if you are a good candidate.

Not to be crass, but I think it's fair to say that the side effects of chemotherapy, radiation, uncontrolled type 2 diabetes, advanced kidney disease/dialysis, etc., are a heck of a lot worse and harder to manage or live with than the side effects associated with AOMs. Knowing that obesity is a HUGE contributor to cancer, DM2, kidney failure, heart disease, etc., why are we only treating advanced

---

[68] "How to Use Mounjaro," Mounjaro website, accessed July 14, 2023, https://www.mounjaro.com/how-to-use-mounjaro.

[69] "Medullary Thyroid Cancer (MTC)," "Rare Endocrine Tumors" section of National Cancer Institute website, published February 27, 2019, www.cancer.gov/pediatric-adult-rare-tumor/rare-tumors/rare-endocrine-tumor/medullary-thyroid-cancer.

diseases instead of using the preventative medication options available? Of course, obesity is not to blame for all of these conditions, but if we could at least lessen the likelihood, especially in those at higher risk, why wouldn't we?

In addition to the physical and medical risks associated with obesity, there are many mental and emotional ones. Many people struggling with obesity aren't just carrying around the physical weight, but the emotional weight too.

I'm a prime example. After years of working on my routine, habits, and mindset around my body and food both with my therapist and my mindset coach, there I was, nearly five years later, struggling and entertaining the idea of going back to restrictive methods. The emotional burden was far worse to deal with on a daily basis than the mild nausea I experienced from Mounjaro. I'll take the latter.

The Stigma Around Weight Loss Medications

I don't fault you if you have a bias toward people who struggle with their weight; fear and criticism around weight gain and loss is so ingrained in our minds due to societal pressures and conditioning. So don't feel guilty or attacked by what I'm about to say; instead, use it as an opportunity to learn.

Here's the truth: If you are against the usage of medication management for weight loss, then there's a good chance you are biased toward people who struggle with obesity.

Some of you may be thinking, *No way, Jamie. I struggle with my weight too, and I am against medication management.* Unfortunately, I am also talking to you. Even those of you who struggle with your weight can have a bias against people who struggle with their weight too. Personal weight struggles and weight bias are *not* mutually exclusive.

And it's okay if that makes you feel some type of way—I'm glad! The whole point of this book is to open your mind to rethinking how you view those with obesity, yourself included.

Obesity is a disease. So, put simply, standing against weight loss medications means standing against people getting help for their disease. Why is one disease more worthy of treatment than another? (Let's really think about that and where the hypocrisy lies.)

The stance against weight loss medications often comes from projecting our own insecurities onto obesity itself. It's great if you don't want to be on medication; no one is saying you have to be. But I'm asking genuinely, why do you care if someone else is? It has *zero* impact on you. (Really let that sink in, because it's true.) It's time for all of us to uproot this stigma and our societal training, as hard as it might be.

The Stigma Within Our Own WLS Community

The number of weight loss surgery patients who are against weight loss medications is interesting, to say the least. With the rise of the GLP-1 usage in the bariatric community, so many bariatric patients have come forward to pass judgment to those going the medications route.

Surgical patients have made and often make harmful remarks, such as the following:

- "Well, if you actually did what you were supposed to after weight loss surgery, you wouldn't need medications."
- "Well, I don't need medication. I've maintained my weight."
- "You should have worked harder after your weight loss surgery, like I did."
- "You're just looking for another quick fix."
- "If you used your tool properly to begin with, you wouldn't need another one."

Talk about the pot calling the freaking kettle black!

The concept that one bariatric patient is "better" than another because they didn't need weight loss medication is a bit absurd. If this is your belief, I'm asking you to take a real hard and close look in the mirror. We are all human beings, and none of us is better than the other. One person may just be struggling more than another and need extra assistance, and that's okay.

As explained earlier, bariatrics is the branch of medicine that deals with the treatment of obesity: this includes weight loss surgery *and* medications. Surgical patients who stand against medication options are against the very thing they chose to do, just via a different method. Call me foolish, but this just doesn't make sense. If this is you, it's time to reevaluate. The best path for you may not be the best path for someone else, but both paths lead to the same destination.

Issues We Are Facing: Shortages and Accessibility

Another rebuttal I've heard to the use of weight loss medications is that they're being taken from diabetics who need them. Let's talk about this for a minute.

We are not "taking" anything from anyone.

Yes, one of the issues with the GLP-1 medications, as a whole, is the accessibility to them due to cost, lack of insurance coverage, and national medication shortages. And yes, GLP-1 and GLP-1/GIP medications were originally intended for diabetes treatment and are FDA approved for type 2 diabetes. But GLP-1 medications such as Saxenda and Wegovy are also now FDA approved as weight loss medications to treat obesity. In addition, Mounjaro, a GLP-1/GIP dual medication FDA approved for DM2, is currently being fast-tracked for FDA approval for obesity treatment. (By the time you read this book, there is a good chance it will already have been approved. Fingers crossed!)

The thing is, so many medications on the market are used to medically treat more than one thing. For example, Lyrica is a medication used to treat generalized anxiety disorder as well as nerve pain for those with diabetic neuropathy and fibromyalgia. You don't see anxiety patients pointing fingers at those with fibromyalgia saying, "You're taking this from us, and we deserve it more than you do."

Diabetes patients absolutely, 100%, should not have to fight to get their medications. So regarding the shortages with Mounjaro, I can understand their frustration with it being prescribed off-label for weight loss. Their experiences are valid. And I think the pharmaceutical companies and physicians prescribing these medications realize just how important it is for people with DM2 to get the medications they need. Heck, I think the people on it for weight loss purposes realize this too. And with the shortages, Lilly, Mounjaro's manufacturing company, has put the proper systems in place to reserve the medication for diabetes patients. They have since changed the terms and conditions on their savings card so that only those with diabetes can opt in. And the majority of insurance companies so far are only approving coverage for Mounjaro for diabetes patients, further reserving the supply for them.

So to be clear, no one is saying that diabetes patients shouldn't have access to their life-saving medications, and while the manufacturing companies are doing their best to restock their supply, they are also putting systems in place to ensure those with DM2 get their medications.

It's also important to note that there are numerous DM2 medications on the market. According to the National Institute for Health, there are currently

> ten classes of orally available pharmacological agents to treat T2DM: 1) sulfonylureas, 2) meglitinides, 3) metformin (a biguanide), 4) thiazolidinediones (TZDs), 5) alpha glucosidase inhibitors, 6) dipeptidyl peptidase IV (DPP-4) inhibitors, 7) bile acid sequestrants, 8) dopamine agonists, 9) sodium-glucose transport protein 2 (SGLT2) inhibitors, and 10) oral glucagon-like peptide 1 (GLP-1) receptor agonists.

> In addition, GLP-1 receptor agonists, dual GLP-1 receptor and GIP receptor agonists, and amylin can be administered by injection.[70]

Note that the last two mentioned are the medications in question for the treatment of obesity. That being said, there are many medication options for those with DM2 (thank goodness!). But there is only one class of medications shown to be effective for weight loss, yielding as much as a 21% loss of total body weight, that can make a substantial difference for those with severe obesity: that's the GLP-1/GIP medications.

I have a hard time believing people would be so angry about this if the Mounjaro was being prescribed off-label for another disease state. For shits and giggles, let's take a minute to imagine Mounjaro is being prescribed off-label for heart disease instead of obesity treatment. Let's pretend that research found that, while Mounjaro is FDA approved for DM2, it was making significant improvements for those with heart disease, leading physicians to prescribe it off-label while pending FDA approval for the miraculous effects it has on improving heart disease.

I wonder if, in that scenario, the world would be pointing fingers at people with heart disease, saying, "How dare you take this medication from diabetes patients who actually need it!" or "You should just work harder at overcoming your disease, because there is a shortage and you don't deserve to be on it." Call me foolish, but I have a *really* hard time believing people with heart disease would be blamed for the shortages. Sounds a hell of a lot like victim blaming to me. Instead, in that scenario, I would imagine the backlash would fall on the shoulders of the manufacturing company or the insurance companies, urging them to restock as quickly as possible to ensure that EVERYONE in need of the medication was able to get it as quickly and affordably as possible.
But again, because it's obesity we are talking about, and society doesn't view it

---

[70] Kenneth R. Feingold, "Oral and Injectable (Non-Insulin) Pharmacological Agents for the Treatment of Type 2 Diabetes," in Feingold et al., eds., *Endotext* [Internet]. South Dartmouth, MA: MDText.com, Inc., 2000–, available at https://www.ncbi.nlm.nih.gov/books/NBK279141/.

as a "real" disease, those with obesity are being BLAMED for getting TREATMENT they DESERVE.

The fact of the matter is supply does not determine need. Plain and simple. And quite frankly, I'm tired of having to explain this to the world.

Cost is also another huge factor when it comes to the accessibility of these medications. Paying out of pocket for the GLP-1 or GLP-1/GIP medications can cost upwards of $1,300 per month out of pocket.

At this point, some insurance companies are covering these medications, especially the ones that are FDA approved for weight loss. However, at this point, the majority of insurance plans don't cover AOMs. And most GLP-1/GIP medications are not covered unless you have a DM2 diagnosis.

Some of the manufacturing companies, such as Novo Nordisk (who manufactures Wegovy) and Lilly (who manufactures Mounjaro) have offered twelve-month savings coupons for those with commercial insurance whose plans do not cover the medications. These savings coupons bring the cost down to about $25 per month for the first year. Which is great, but what happens when the year is over?

As of January 1, 2023, Lilly changed the terms and conditions on their savings card for Mounjaro. Now only those with an active DM2 diagnosis are able to be on it for $25 per month. Those without a DM2 diagnosis can still opt in, but the savings card only saves about $500, making the out-of-pocket cost around $800 or more per month—which still is not accessible or affordable for most people. On one hand, I do think it is good they have some policies in place in order to reserve medications for those with DM2. Like I mentioned before, people with diabetes should not have to fight for their medications. But on the other hand, it continues to limit those with obesity and comorbidities who are also deserving of treatment.

There are additional cost concerns with the medications. One concern is that this new demand for these medications will drive up the costs for people with diabetes, limiting their access.

I do agree that this is a concern and problem. But it's not a problem people with obesity created or had a hand in. This is a systemic and nationwide healthcare issue. Healthcare in the United States never should have been a for-profit system. That right there is the root of the issues at hand. It's not the burden of the patients to bear that they need a medication their physician is prescribing to them, diabetes or not.

I'm not a politician, and I won't pretend to be for even a second. I don't have the answers to how to implement universal healthcare, and it's not a problem I think any one of us could singularly tackle. But as a practitioner and patient, I firmly believe this is why we are having the problems we are having. Because of the systems above us. Not because of the fault of the patients.

If the World Viewed Obesity as a Disease, This Wouldn't Even Be Up for Debate

Obesity is a disease. One that deserves treatment. (Wow, how many times can I say that in this book?) If we have a groundbreaking medical treatment for obesity, why shouldn't people who struggle be allowed to receive it?

It's because, once again, our world does not view obesity as a disease worthy of being treated. Our society simply views it as a moral failing. As laziness. As a matter of simply "trying harder." Why is obesity the only disease that seems to be on the receiving end of these comments?

Because, if we are really going to be honest here, many diseases can be prevented or treated with lifestyle management. Eating well, exercising, getting enough sleep, etc. can reduce your risk of DM2, heart disease, stroke, high cholesterol, high blood pressure, and cancer. But you don't walk up to a stroke victim and say, "Well, you should just try harder. Get up and work for it, you lazy POS." No, that never happens. So WHY does this happen for those with obesity?

And in case the world has forgotten, if you treat obesity, you are prematurely treating and preventing the likelihood of those other aforementioned diseases from arising! From a public-health standpoint, why aren't we more vigorously treating obesity early to avoid all the other complications that come along with it?

But no, why would we do the logical thing when we can just continue to shame people with obesity, as we have always done?

The world tells us to lose weight. They tell us we aren't healthy. They tell us to do whatever we need to, to grit through it, to no longer be "fat."

But when we do just that, when we find an incredible treatment option, we are told, "Not that way, you selfish and lazy asshole." This may sound harsh, but we know it's true. And I'm just so tired of people who struggle with their weight being continually shamed and blamed from so many angles for seeking treatment.

All I want is for one person to make it make sense. I'll wait.

Bite-Sized Recap

- GLP-1s are meant to be taken long term.
- It certainly is possible to come off of the medications, if you want or need to, but I think it's important to understand that most people will gain the weight back if and when they do.
- The most common side effects reported are nausea, constipation, and/or diarrhea. These primary side effects are easily managed for most.
- If you are against the usage of medication management for weight loss, then there's a good chance you are biased toward people who struggle with obesity, even if you yourself struggle with your weight.
- Unfortunately, there is a lot of judgment within the surgical bariatric community pertaining to others utilizing these medications.
- Standing against weight loss medications means standing against people getting help for their disease. It is not a competition amongst varying diseases and who is most "deserving" of treatment. Any and all who struggle with any disease deserve treatment.
- Manufacturer shortages, insurance coverage, and other accessibility issues are the largest barriers for people obtaining these medications.
- Supply does not determine need.

For journal prompts and resources related to this chapter be sure to head to www.thesleeveddietitian.com/easy.

Chapter 6
But Isn't It Healthy?

health·y
/helTHē/
adjective
1. in good health.
"I feel fit and healthy."

What I Quickly Realized About Healthy Eating

I thought I knew everything I needed to know about nutrition. Well, maybe not everything. But I felt like I, of all people, would be the "perfect" weight loss surgery candidate, because I already "knew what I was doing."

Until I sat down for my first nutrition session with my own bariatric dietitian.

Let me tell you, I was humbled real quick.

So much of what I knew about nutrition simply didn't apply to a bariatric lifestyle. I was blown away by the things I would need to omit from my diet in order to prepare for surgery. During the pre-op stages, most WLS patients are encouraged to start making the habit changes in the three to six months leading up to their surgery, since it can be so hard to get a grasp on what is and is not "okay" after surgery.

Habits I felt were "healthy" (and by general nutrition standards were) had to go out the window. I remember when I first learned that I had to give up my seltzer water; I was dumbfounded. *But it's sugar-free! But it's calorie free! But it's such a better choice than sugar-sweetened beverages! It's basically just water!* All of these thoughts ran through my head, and if you're new to the surgery world, you probably are having the same reaction.

Bariatric nutrition is considered a "specialty" in the nutrition world. Foods that are totally healthy and encouraged for the general population aiming to lose weight (without surgery) either aren't recommended or reasonable after weight loss surgery.

In Chapter 9, I'm going to share more with you about why some things aren't recommended after weight loss surgery. But for now, I'm going to share with you why some nutrition habits that are viewed as healthy simply aren't reasonable after weight loss surgery. I'm also going to touch on why foods society views as "unhealthy" are actually encouraged post-op.

Wellness Culture and All Its Confusion

I think it's only fair to bring light to the fact that nutrition, in general, is confusing. I say this often: nutrition is a SCIENCE not an OPINION. But yet everyone has an opinion. And how could you not? Nutrition is so personal. Nutrition is cultural. It's generational. It's societal. It's social. It's emotional. It's so individualized, and yet the world fails to see the nuances. So how do we take what science tells us about nutrition, how food works in our bodies, or how our bodies process and react to foods, and still hold space for everyone's unique take on what does and does not work for them?

I think both diet and wellness culture play a big role in this. There is more pushback right now in the social space when it comes to diet culture. As more people become more educated and recognize the toxicities that lie within fad diets and harmful trends, more people are rejecting the restrictive diet mentality. Which is fantastic, might I add.

But on that same token, there has been a huge uprising in wellness culture. According to registered dietitian and author of *The Wellness Trap* and *Anti-Diet*,

Christy Harrison defines wellness culture as "a set of values that equates wellness with moral goodness, and posits certain behaviors—and a certain type of body—as the path to achieving that supposed rectitude."[71]

I'd like for you to pause for a minute and ask yourself this: when you hear the term "wellness culture," and its definition, what comes to mind?

For me, when I think of wellness culture, I picture very lean women posting on social media in their Lululemon leggings, stretching on a yoga mat. I picture them sharing their cold-pressed green juice and eating beautiful, organic, plant-based meals. I see them drinking lemon water out of a pretty little mason jar. I see them sharing their beliefs of the beauties of "clean eating." I think of the posts that tell you not to eat processed foods, because they have seed oils or they "cause inflammation" and are bad for your "gut health." But perhaps this image that comes to my mind is a bit biased or stereotypical, based on my own thoughts and experiences (both professionally and personally), and perhaps your connotation of wellness culture is different from mine.

I'm not saying any of these things are bad. They're not. In fact, a lot of these messages are rooted in the science of nutrition. I don't think anyone is about to argue that whole foods, filled with fiber, drinking lots of water, and getting movement in could possibly be bad. However, over time, I believe these messages have been taken to extremes, and now what we have are a lot of confusing and skewed messages to those watching from afar.

A good example is the use of the term "clean eating." God, I hate this phrase. I may ruffle some feathers here, and I hate to break it to you, but there is no such thing as "clean eating." Unless you dropped your food on the floor for more than five seconds, or your food has mold growing on it, chances are, it's clean! Now, I know that what people who use this term mean is foods that are in their

[71] Christy Harrison, "Wellness Culture," christyharrison.com website, accessed July 14, 2023, https://christyharrison.com/wellness-culture#:~:text=Wellness%20culture%20is%20a%20set,to%20achieving%20that%20supposed%20rectitude.

whole form and minimally processed. But the message this sends ultimately is that some foods are "good" to eat whereas others are "bad," which is a black-and-white way of thinking our society truly needs to get out of.

Foods are not good or bad; they are just different. Some may serve us on our journey or in hitting our goals and others may not (as I'm going to share with you soon). It's also important to note that each and every person's goals when it comes to obtaining their ideal version of health is going to be different. What's even wilder to me is the people who use these terms are often trying to sell you something beyond just good old healthy eating tips. More often than not, they're trying to sell you a green juice or a protein blend of some kind that is "full of clean ingredients." The real kicker here? Those protein powders and powdered greens are still heavily processed! What I'm trying to get at is that strict health protocols and wellness culture are pretty much the same packages as diet culture, just wrapped in a different bow. And while the components may be a bit different, the delivery and end message seem to be the same: *eat this way and buy the thing I'm selling, or you're doing it wrong and can't possibly be healthy like me.*

And just like with diet culture, in wellness culture, there are a LOT of buzz words and phrases. There are also a lot of scare tactics and lots of fearmongering. Whenever you see someone praising "clean eating" or "eat this food to reduce inflammation" or "do this for a metabolic reset," just know that, even if they are well-intentioned, these phrases are projecting wellness culture and portraying an unrealistic standard of eating that most people are not able to be consistent with. And if that's the case, even if some of these things are healthy, if you can't stick to them, then they aren't really helping at the end of the day, are they?

Some Nuances Between General Nutrition and Bariatric Nutrition

The things I'm discussing below are not "bad." They just aren't always applicable to people after weight loss surgery, no matter how much society says they are what's healthiest. There are many nuances when it comes to this topic, but I've chosen to focus on some of the most common ones I see.

Eating Lots of Fruits, Veggies, and Whole Foods

As much as most people want to add these things in after surgery, so many cannot. The number one reason this is so hard for WLS patients is because so many simply just do not tolerate fruits and vegetables after surgery.

Fruits and vegetables are fantastic because they add lots of water, fiber, and nutrients to your diet. They help with digestion, and they help keep you fuller longer. For bariatric patients, specifically, whole-food sources, fruits, and vegetables help to "maximize your restriction"; in other words, use your bariatric tool in a way that lets you fill up your bariatric belly with foods that are going to allow you to feel fullness most readily.

All great things! But where the nuance, or exception, comes in is when bariatric patients don't tolerate these foods. While highly fibrous foods are fantastic, for someone getting bariatric surgery (or any gastrointestinal surgery, for that matter), these foods can become irritants and may not settle well in their new stomach. These foods are hard to break down, and some aren't able to break them down the way they were before. This can cause patients to feel very sick and uncomfortable. The most common thing I hear from patients is that these foods feel "stuck" after they eat them, like they won't move through from their esophagus to their stomach properly and instead just "sit heavy." Personally, I can relate to this feeling too.

I was having a discussion with a weight loss surgery patient of mine who is in one of my group coaching programs, and she was sharing with me how much she truly misses vegetables. She lives in New Mexico, where she has access to farmers markets that have an abundance of fresh produce that she loves. She shared with me on a call that she struggles so much with eating produce, because it makes her sick and not feel well. She knows she's supposed to be adding more fruits and vegetables to her plate to help keep her fuller longer, but despite knowing this and wanting to do this, she can't. Her body just does not tolerate them, no matter how she cooks or prepares them.

And that's okay. We found a way to work around it. Instead, I supported her in finding some other solutions. In addition to taking her vitamins consistently to get her micronutrient needs met, we also came up with a plan for her to add more complex carbs such as beans, lentils, whole grains, oatmeal, and brown rice to her routine so that she is able to get more fiber and extra nutrition into her diet. And that, for her, right now, is the healthiest thing she can do. But it's taking ongoing work for her to accept that this IS her version of healthy, since she continues to feel like she's not "doing good enough," because she isn't able to add the things everyone tells her she should add.

Drinking Plain Water

Water. The most basic and most important nutrient that the body needs. It's wild that after weight loss surgery, drinking water becomes hard. With limited stomach capacity, rules surrounding drinking (which I'll get into in the next chapter), and changes in body signals and sensations, drinking water can be such a challenge.

Many bariatric patients report a decreased sensation of thirst after weight loss surgery, and many will say that they no longer feel the urge or need to drink. I can relate to this very much. Prior to weight loss surgery, I would easily drink a gallon of water per day, no problem. Now? Now I have to put timers and alarms on my phone, even more than five years post-op, to remind myself to drink water, since my body doesn't seem to want to give me that internal cue anymore. I have yet to find research to back the reason for this, but if I had to make an educated guess, I would assume it must have something to do with our hormone signaling to the brain. The hypothalamus regulates hunger and thirst. Ghrelin, the hunger hormone, is the hormone that regulates hunger, whereas **angiotensin II (AngII)** is the main hormone that regulates thirst.[72]

[72] David E. Leib et al., "Thirst," Current Biology 26, no. 24 (December 2016): R1260–1265, https://

Given the changes in ghrelin-signaling post WLS, thirst signals may also be affected post-op.

In addition to these struggles above, another one of the most common things I hear from bariatric patients is "Plain water makes me nauseous." Many have shared with me that plain water can even make them vomit. I'm not going to lie, I'm not sure I would have believed this one, but I have also experienced this since surgery. I used to LOVE plain water. There really was nothing better than a cold glass of water with some lemon or lime juice squeezed into it. And while this "water nausea" effect doesn't happen to everyone after bariatric surgery (so if you're pre-op and reading this, please know that although this is a possibility, it's not universal), it does seem to happen quite a bit.

It's still unclear exactly why this happens, as there's not a lot of data or science to support the first hand accounts given by patients. However, according to The Center for Bariatrics at Bailey Medical Center in Owasso, Oklahoma, this phenomenon may be due to potential dehydration, electrolyte imbalance, the difference in acidity in the stomach or changes to the stomach as part of the surgery process.[73] Personally, hearing the theory of the changes in stomach acidity seems to make sense.

Even if you're like me, and you struggle with drinking water after surgery, or you need timers to remind you to drink on your phone, I'm happy to report that most WLS patients do ultimately find ways to get their water in, as it's SO important to avoid the consequences of dehydration. In order to make sure this doesn't happen and to make water a priority, you may need to think more strategically around your hydration habits.

MY TOP 3 TIPS FOR STAYING HYDRATED POST BARIATRIC SURGERY:

1. Put timers on your phone: make sure you remember to sip your water

www.ncbi.nlm.nih.gov/pmc/articles/PMC5957508/.

[73] "Water Nausea after Bariatric Surgery," Center for Bariatrics at Bailey Medical Center website, accessed July 14, 2023, https://baileybariatrics.com/blog/water-nausea-after-bariatric-surgery#:~:text=If%20you%20aren't%20tolerating,plain%20water%20isn't%20tolerated.

consistently throughout the day and in between meals and snacks.

2. Have a water bottle with you at all times: believe it or not, having a water bottle close by can help you remember to drink enough.
3. Flavor your water: using different sugar-free flavors and water enhancers can really help people stay hydrated, especially since oftentimes, flavored water seems to minimize nausea, for whatever reason.

"But Jamie, artificial sweeteners are AWFUL for you! Don't you know that?"

Artificial sweeteners have a terrible reputation, especially within wellness culture. There's a lot of misinformation and personal viewpoints that contribute to this. I would like to start off by saying that I think everyone is entitled to personal feelings about certain foods, and if you feel like something isn't suited for you or your lifestyle, then you shouldn't have it. This is not me trying to change your mind. But as I mentioned in the beginning of this chapter, nutrition is a science. And thus far, the science sides with the conclusion that sugar substitutes are safe to consume.

Technically, the proper name for sugar substitutes are "non-nutritive sweeteners," meaning sweeteners both of natural and artificial origin that do not add calories to your intake.

Currently, there are six artificial sweeteners that are FDA approved. These artificial sweeteners include: saccharin, aspartame, acesulfame potassium (acesulfame-K, or Ace-K), sucralose, neotame, and advantame. For the naturally occurring, plant-based, non-nutritive sweeteners, the FDA generally recognizes stevia, luo han guo (also known as "monk fruit"), and thaumatin as safe.[74]

According to the National Cancer Institute, as of 2023, there is NOT a definitive link between artificial sweeteners and cancer in people.[75] They explain that

---

[74] "Artificial Sweeteners and Cancer," "Cancer Causes and Prevention: Risk Factors: Diet" section of National Cancer Institute website, last updated January 12, 2023, https://www.cancer.gov/about-cancer/causes-prevention/risk/diet/artificial-sweeteners-fact-sheet.

[75] National Cancer Institute, "Artificial Sweeteners."

this assumption generally comes from early studies done between the 1970s and 80s, in which rats developed bladder cancer after being given sweeteners called cyclamate and saccharin. Cyclamate was banned from the US, and as of the year 2000, mechanistic studies that examined how saccharin works in the human body versus a rat's found the substance's contribution to bladder cancer in rats does not apply to humans.[76]

However, new fear has been sparked regarding the sweetener aspartame. In July of 2023 it was reported that WHO's cancer research agency, the International Agency for Research on Cancer (IARC), has declared aspartame a possible carcinogen.[77] Now, I know this verbiage may sound scary, but I want you to truly understand what this means. While it's easy to jump to the conclusion that aspartame causes cancer, that is not the case, and I want you to be aware of how fearmongering from the wellness industry is skewing things, yet again.

According to the Natural Institute of Health, the term "carcinogen" refers to anything that is capable of causing cancer, including substances, organisms, and agents both naturally occurring in the environment (such as ultraviolet rays in the sun) and man-made (such as cigarette smoke).[78]

With rising fear surrounding aspartame as a carcinogen, one important detail that many are not taking into account is the classification of carcinogens in which the IARC opted to include aspartame.

To put that in context, the IARC uses four different carcinogenic classifications. The groups are as follows:

- Group 1: Carcinogenic to humans

---

[76] National Cancer Institute, "Artificial Sweeteners."
[77] Daryl Austin, "Aspartame is a Possible Carcinogen, WHO Says. Should You Stop Drinking Diet Soda?," "Diet and Fitness" section of *Today* website, published July 3, 2023, https://www.today.com/health/diet-fitness/aspartame-carcinogen-diet-soda-rcna92376.
[78] "Carcinogen," About Genomics: Educational Resources, Talking Glossary of Genomic and Genetic Terms, National Human Genome Research Institute, last updated July 14, 2023, https://www.genome.gov/genetics-glossary/Carcinogen.

- Group 2A: Probably carcinogenic to humans
- Group 2B: Possibly carcinogenic to humans
- Group 3: Not classifiable as to its carcinogenicity to humans[79]

To give you a better understanding of Group 2B carcinogens, the list includes aloe vera, pickled vegetables, and drycleaning your clothes. To give you an even better understanding, Group 2A, which is more likely to be carcinogenic to humans, includes working night shifts and red meat consumption.[80] Alcoholic beverages are a Group 1 classification.

The American Cancer Society states:

> It's important to know that **IARC classifications are based on the strength of the evidence of whether something can cause cancer in humans, not how likely it is to cause cancer**. The Group 2B classification is the third highest out of 4 levels, and it is generally used either when there is limited, but not convincing, evidence for cancer in humans, or when there is convincing evidence for cancer in lab animals, but not both.[81]

Just because something is on the IARC classifications list doesn't mean it automatically will lead to cancer in humans. Does this mean you shouldn't ever eat red meat, walk outside under the sun, or work the night shift? No, absolutely not. We can consume or be exposed to all of these things without it automatically resulting in cancer.

And while we don't know exactly how much aspartame potentially could be

---

[79] "Agents Classified by the IARC Monographs, Volumes 1–134," "Classifications" page on International Agency for Research on Cancer website, last updated July 14, 2023, https://monographs.iarc.who.int/agents-classified-by-the-iarc/.

[80] "List of Classifications: Agents Classified by the IARC Monographs, Volumes 1–134," Classifications, International Agency for Research on Cancer, last updated July 14, 2023, https://monographs.iarc.who.int/list-of-classifications/.

[81] Emphasis added. "Aspartame and Cancer Risk," "Cancer Risk and Prevention: Chemicals" page on American Cancer Society website, last updated July 13, 2023, https://www.cancer.org/cancer/risk-prevention/chemicals/aspartame.html.

"too much," according to the Food and Drug Administration (FDA) the acceptable daily intake suggestion is approximately 50 milligrams per kilogram of body weight per day.[82] To give you a frame of reference, for someone who is 150 pounds, that would be approximately 17 12-oz cans of Diet Coke every day.[83]

What is interesting though, which the National Cancer Institute also notes, is that some suggest that artificial sweeteners have an association with obesity, as it's been previously thought that artificial sweeteners may raise blood sugar and increase "real" sugar cravings. However, they explained that a "systematic review and meta-analysis of 17 randomized controlled trials in adults found that substituting low- and no-calorie sweetened beverages for sugar-sweetened beverages was associated with small improvements in body weight."[84]

I think what is so interesting about this is that the only real concern ever linked to artificial sweeteners in relation to cancer was the thought that they might be linked to obesity—because *obesity* is what was a risk factor for cancer, not the artificial sweeteners itself.

In the bariatric community, the most important thing yet again is going back to treating obesity, especially to avoid these serious comorbidities. Which is why, I believe, if having artificial sweeteners in your diet allows you to get your fluids in after surgery and stay away from sugar-sweetened items and beverages that are known to contribute to obesity rates, then the artificial sweeteners are a far better option.[85]

So basically, what I'm saying is you can all keep your Crystal Light and sugar-free Gatorade. If that's what you like, what you tolerate, what keeps you hydrated, and what allows you to stay consistent with hitting your goals post-op,

---

[82] American Cancer Society, "Aspartame and Cancer Risk."
[83] Austin, "Aspartame Is a Possible Carcinogen."
[84] "Artificial Sweeteners and Cancer," "Diet" section of National Cancer Institute website, last updated January 12, 2023. https://www.cancer.gov/about-cancer/causes-prevention/risk/diet/artificial-sweeteners-fact-sheet#do-artificial-sweeteners-contribute-toplay-a-role-in-obesity.
[85] National Cancer Institute, "Artificial Sweeteners."

then I see no reason to stop.

Avoiding Processed Foods

Ahhh yes, another controversial topic of conversation. Hold on to your seats, wellness culture heroes, because yes, I am going to firmly say that it is okay, and often even *encouraged*, for bariatric patients to have processed foods in their post-op routine. GASP! No, not the processed foods! How dare I, a registered dietitian, make such a suggestion!

I hope by now you are picking up on my sarcasm and humor. Just like with artificial sweeteners, there are a lot of mixed feelings and opinions around processed foods. I really do not believe that any dietitian is going to tell you to eat all processed foods. Nor would I, or my colleagues, encourage you to make up the majority of your diet from processed foods. But the reality is, not all processed foods are "bad." And if we are talking about the general population here for a moment, processed foods are necessary for the average family to put food on the table. Not only are processed foods shelf-stable, they also are more affordable.

You will learn in the next chapter that, as a bariatric patient, getting your protein needs met is of the utmost importance to avoid malnutrition. Sometimes, in order to get those needs met, having protein-fortified food options such as protein shakes, protein bars, or other protein-based products are a necessary part of a healthy bariatric lifestyle. All of these protein-fortified options are processed. That doesn't mean they are bad. They are actually so important for most patients to have on hand.

And this is where wellness culture can become so toxic, as it is, quite honestly, riddled with privilege. Wellness culture disavows non-White food in many instances, leading people to believe that their traditional and cultural foods are "not healthy" simply because they aren't from Western or European traditions. Wellness culture rhetoric will also have you believe that if you don't grow your own food, buy farm-fresh and organic everything, or prepare all of your meals from scratch, then you are "lazy" or you don't care about your family's health, which couldn't be further from the truth. Most people are doing their best to just stay afloat and put food on the table and provide a decent meal for themselves and their family.

And as for me? Well, quite frankly, I hate cooking. I find it stressful, messy, and overall unenjoyable. It feels like just another chore. And as a full-time entrepreneur with a never-ending to-do list and ADHD, it's unlikely that at the end of my 10+ hour day, I'm making an entire meal from scratch every night. And I don't even have the responsibility of having littles to feed on top of it, so I can't even imagine that additional stress.

Since the beginning of my journey, I have relied on convenience items, whether that be ready-made options or partially prepared options. Especially when I was in my dietetic internship and juggling school and clinical rotations. Most nights, my dinner looks like me throwing some Perdue low-carb chicken tenders in the air fryer, pairing it with some microwaved frozen broccoli and low-sugar or sugar-free honey mustard for dipping, and calling it a day. And you know what? Sometimes good enough is good enough. It checks the boxes. I have my protein. I have a lower carb option. I pair it with some easy steamed vegetables. It's balanced. It's convenient. It's "bariatric friendly." And most importantly? I like it enough to eat it often and be consistent. I can tell you first-hand that having a mentality of consistency, over perfection, has served me so much better than putting pressure on myself to "eat clean" ever did.

Shame and Guilt

Shame and guilt runs strong amongst bariatric patients. So many people already feel shamed for having surgery because of all the stigmas. To top it off, it can be really hard when they feel like they had surgery and are still doing it "wrong" or having foods that society says is "bad." I can't tell you how often someone tells me, "I know it's bad that I have to have Crystal Light, but without it, I just can't get my water in," or "I know I should be eating more veggies, but they just hurt my stomach when I eat them," or "I feel like I'm ruining this journey by not being healthy."

And if this is you, and you can relate, what I want you to know is not any one habit or food can deem your health routine "bad." If something works for you, allows you to get adequate nutrition, and is able to sustain you physically and emotionally, is it really "bad" just because society and the media tells you it is? What makes up your entire routine and how all the pieces come together is what will truly make the biggest impact on your health and your goals on your weight loss surgery journey.

The Main Point

I want to make sure I'm being very clear here: I'm not saying that bariatric patients should just never drink plain water or eat fruits and veggies on their journey and that they should just have lots of processed foods. Not even a little bit. In fact, in the next few chapters, I'm going to teach you how to implement many of the bariatric dos and don'ts. But what I am saying is that, sometimes, the stigmas that are projected by wellness culture and seen in society as the epitome of health are not always realistic for bariatric patients. And it genuinely hurts my heart to see people feel like they are "failing" because they are not meeting society's ideal health standards. If you're reading this, and that resonates with you, I want you to know, the only people's standards you need to meet are *your own*, and the standards you've outlined with your weight loss surgery team.

Nutrition is not one-size-fits-all. Bariatric patient or not, we all have unique needs, challenges, routines, responsibilities, life hurdles, and circumstances. Deciding what's healthiest for each person is up to interpretation. It's not black and white. And I firmly believe that one of the most important factors in determining outcomes for bariatric patients is their ability to be consistent in the habits that will serve them long term. So if that means having some Diet

Snapple or throwing some low-carb chicken nuggies in the air fryer and microwaving some rice and veggies, so be it.

Is having a diet high in refined sugar and candy recommended? No, not usually. But, again, you need to look at each person. For some people who are in eating disorder recovery, regularly having processed sugars in their diet to overcome food fears and triggers is encouraged. For others, even those trying to lose weight, having a serving of candy each day may be what they need to stay consistent and make really awesome choices the rest of the time to hit their goals.

Just because something is labeled by society as "healthy" doesn't mean it's going to help you hit your goals. You can walk into any Whole Foods Market and head straight to their bakery aisle and choose the "healthiest," all organic, almond flour, coconut sugar, etc. brand of cookies; but at the end of the day, it's still a cookie, and if you overeat it, like anything else, it's going to cause weight gain. But again, if your goal isn't weight loss or you have celiac disease (a gluten allergy, where you may need wheat flour substitutes), then maybe it is going to be the healthier option. The nuances go on and on.

Everyone's definition of what's healthy will vary. What every person needs to be consistent to achieve their health and weight goals will also be different. But at the end of the day, nutrition does boil down to a science. It's just how you take that with you and apply it to your own life. Especially after weight loss surgery. There is no right or wrong way to approach your lifestyle after surgery, as long as what you are doing is working for YOU and YOUR family.

That's what really matters.

Bite-Sized Recap

- Nutrition is a science, not an opinion. Yet everyone has their own opinion—shaped by their own life experiences—on what is healthy, all of which are valid and important.
- Nutrition, by and large, is confusing. And there are many mixed messages about what is and is not healthy.
- Wellness culture is not attainable for everyone and is projecting unrealistic expectations that do not leave room for nuances in one's own journey, which can result in unnecessary shame and guilt.
- Bariatric nutrition is not the same as general nutrition, and oftentimes the things bariatric patients must do to hit their nutrient needs and maintain their health goes against what most of society would deem as "healthy."
- The idea of health is going to be different for everyone, depending on their goals and life circumstances. Space should be held for each individual situation.

For journal prompts and resources related to this chapter be sure to head to www.thesleeveddietitian.com/easy.

Chapter 7
Nutrition After Weight Loss Surgery

nu·tri·tion

/no͞oˈtriSH(ə)n/

noun

1. the process of providing or obtaining the food necessary for health and growth

"a guide to good nutrition"

2. the branch of science that deals with nutrients and nutrition, particularly in humans

"She relied on the guidance of her dietitian for nutrition support."

Nutrition Is What You WILL eat, Not What You WON'T

I'm not sure who needs to hear this, but nutrition (and your overall "diet") is not the same thing as "dieting." In terms of nutrition, when we talk about diet, we are referring to the overall makeup of your eating habits and routine.

The goal in life, even after weight loss surgery, is not to eat as little as possible for as long as possible. The goal is to nourish your body, feed it, and give it all the nutrients it needs to thrive and function.

As silly as it sounds, I don't think I realized this myself until I was fully immersed in my undergraduate dietetics program. The whole role of a registered dietitian, I learned, is to FEED people—whether that be someone who we need to feed through a feeding tube because they're sick in the hospital or someone working on weight loss. The whole point is to support LIFE, and we cannot do that if we don't eat, and we cannot do that if we don't eat properly.

My whole life, I was always told to eat less. As someone who always struggled with weight, eating less was always the goal. My young and naive adolescent brain couldn't have possibly known better. Less equaled weight loss, which equaled health. That was the only equation I knew.

When you grow up continually shamed for your weight and for the foods you are eating, it's easy to associate eating with shame. In many people's brains, even if it's subconsciously, eating is usually labeled as "bad."

But you need to eat. You always need to nourish yourself. And I'd like to teach you how to do that after weight loss surgery.

Portions and Diet Progression After WLS

Everyone's portions are going to look different after weight loss surgery. It can be really hard to conceptualize this when you first have surgery, and sometimes, the amount of food you're able to eat isn't what you thought it'd be. It can also be really hard to wrap your head around what your portions should or will look like if you are comparing what you are eating to what others are eating. And this is because surgery isn't one-size-fits-all, and everyone is going to be able to eat different amounts of food after it.

Why Everyone's Portions Are Different

Did you know that after weight loss surgery, everyone's stomach size (or pouch size, as it's also referred to) is going to be different? It's true. Every surgeon cuts and performs surgery slightly differently. Some surgeons make patients' pouches extra small, while others are more liberal with the pouch size—hence there being so much variability in how much food each person can eat afterwards.

When surgeons perform surgery, specifically when they perform the VSG, they use what is called a "bougie" or a "bougie gauge" to determine the pouch size. A bougie is

> a measuring device developed in France that is in the form of a long, flexible tube and used in gastric sleeve surgery to guide surgeons when dividing the stomach. The tube is inserted into the patient's mouth and then guided through the food pipe and the stomach to the pylorus (part of the stomach). The bougie helps surgeons create a bulge, which is then used to guide the stapler and create a stomach sleeve."[86]

Bougie sizes typically range from 32–60 French.[87] French (Fr) is the unit of measurement for the bougie. For example, the bougie size a surgeon may choose might be "32Fr." The French unit of measurement is equal to ⅓ of a millimeter (mm).[88] For a frame of reference, a 40Fr bougie is approximately ½ of an inch. Surgeons usually choose the sizing based on their preferences as well as their patients' needs and goals.

Ultimately, this is going to change how much you are able to eat, so if you can eat more or less than what you expected, please know that everyone's pouch size and restriction is going to be different.

Weight vs. Volume and How to Figure Out Your Portions

When it comes to determining and measuring your portions after WLS, there is some debate about whether your portions should be accounted for in weight or volume. Personally, I've always weighed my food on a food scale and used ounces as the metric by which to measure my intake. However, other surgical centers and dietitians will suggest using cup sizes to account for volume

---

[86] Ravi Rao, "Vertical Sleeve Gastrectomy,: Answering 4 FAQ's on Bougie Size," Perth Surgical and Bariatrics website blog, https://www.perthsurgicalbariatrics.com.au/vertical-sleeve-gastrectomy-answering-4-faqs-on-bougie-size/#:~:text=1.,surgeons%20when%20dividing%20the%20stomach.
[87] Abdelkader Hawasli et al., "Early Effects of Bougie Size on Sleeve Gastrectomy Ooutcome," *American Journal of Surgery* 209, no. 3: 473–477, https://www.americanjournalofsurgery.com/article/S0002-9610(14)00603-5/fulltext,
[88] Ron Elli, "What's My Bougie Size? Gastric Sleeve Surgery Outcome," Mexico Bariatric Center website, published June 5, 2021, https://mexicobariatriccenter.com/what-is-my-bougie-size-gastric-sleeve-surgery/.

or weight. I really don't believe that there is a right or wrong way to do this, but the one caveat is that some foods will weigh significantly less on the scale while still adding up in volume. For example, 2 ounces of chicken, which is rather dense, is going to look very different than 2 ounces of popcorn, which is very light on the food scale, so that is something to keep in mind.

Some people do get super particular with this after weight loss surgery. I often see people weighing out all of their food into grams for the purpose of figuring out the exact calories or macros in everything, for meticulous tracking and logging of food. To each their own, but I personally don't suggest this strategy, as it often becomes obsessive. I'll discuss calories, tracking, and more of my thoughts on this a bit later.

I also have a lot of clients who—because the counting can become obsessive and triggering—not only don't track their food, but also don't weigh or measure. For these patients, I usually suggest simply purchasing small bowls and appetizer plates (usually 6" in diameter) and using the smaller plate settings as a way to gauge their potions using my meal plate method.

Again, there isn't a right or wrong way to approach bariatric surgery. There are multiple strategies or techniques you can use to make sure you are hitting your goals and focusing on your portions and intake.

Average Portion Sizes and Diet Progression

Despite knowing that everyone's stomach size is different after weight loss surgery, there are some general averages and suggestions for what your intake might look like as you move through the diet phases/progression. Typically, most people will start off eating around ¼ to ½ cup of food at a time in the first three to six months after surgery, and they will continue to increase and progress from there until reaching 1 to 1 ½ cups at a time for the long term. *Please keep in mind that every surgery center has slightly different post-op diet requirements, so this is not a prescription or a meal plan, but rather a way of showing you what your meals/post-op diet might look like on average.*

Average Portion Sizes and Diet Progression

Post-Op Stage	**Diet Type**	**Average Portion Suggestion at a Time**
1–2 Weeks Post-Op	Liquid Consistency	Usually suggested to aim for 64 oz fluid + 60 g protein via protein shakes
2–3 Weeks Post-Op	Pureed Consistency	1–3 oz ¼ cup
3–4 Weeks Post-Op	Soft Food Consist-ency	1–3 oz ¼ cup
1–3 Months Post-Op	Solid Foods	3 oz ¼ cup
3–6 Months Post-Op	Solid Foods	4-6 oz ¼–½ cup
6–12 Months Post-Op	Solid Foods	6-8 oz ½1- cup
12–24 Months Post-Op	Solid Foods	8-12 oz 1–1 ½ cups
2+ Years and Be-yond	Solid Foods	Continue to increase as needed long term, although many will keep to 1–1 ½ cups long term.

Now, again, this may vary from person to person. But the main point is, over time, you will be able to eat more food and increase your portion sizes. As you continue to heal, the swelling in your pouch will go down and your new stomach will regain some of that elasticity. It doesn't mean you've "stretched" your pouch or "ruined your surgery." It simply means you are right on target with healing and progressing.

I was very fortunate that when going through the required pre-op appointments with my dietitian, she explained to me that this would happen. But I know that's not the case for everyone. So in case no one has ever told you this, let me pass along her message to all of you: If you do not increase your portions over time, you will starve. Four ounces or a ½ cup of food is NOT healthy or sustainable for anyone long term. Eating more is a GOOD thing and should happen. Again, the purpose of WLS isn't to "diet," restrict, or eat as little as possible for as long as possible. The goal is to get back to a "normal," healthful diet ("diet" meaning your food routine, not a fad diet) that you can sustain throughout your life.

And it's okay if you eat less than what's listed here. It's also okay if you can eat more than what's listed here. I always tell my clients that while, yes, portions do matter, it's the QUALITY of your meals and food habits that matter a heck of a lot more than the QUANTITY of your food intake.

The Bariatric Meal Plate Method

Most bariatric dietitians use some variation of the meal plate method to teach nutrition after weight loss surgery. Above is the image of the version of this meal plate method I teach my clients and members using my Bariatric Breakthrough Method®. The meal plate method generally mimics the MyPlate, which is the visual to represent the official Dietary Guidelines for Americans. This visual replaced the old food pyramid suggestions.[89]

[89] MyPlate website, US Department of Agriculture, accessed July 14, 2023, https://www.myplate.gov/.

The Bariatric Breakthrough® Meal Plate Method

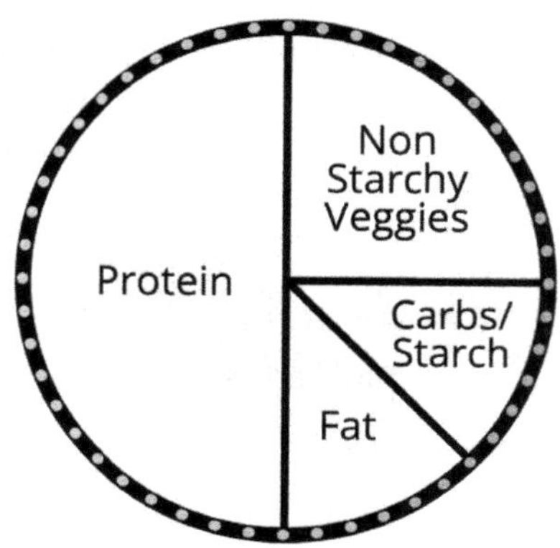

Graphic of the Bariatric Breakthrough Meal Plate Method. Circle representing a plate that is divided into four sections with ½ of the plate protein, ¼ of the plate non-starchy veggies, ⅛ of the plate carbs/starch, and ⅛ of the plate fat.

The reason bariatric patients need their own adjusted meal plate approach is because, with stomach space being so small compared to the average person, certain nutrients take priority over others in order to avoid malnutrition as well as to make sure you are filling your pouch and utilizing your tool properly and maintaining the integrity of your tool long term. It's not just the portion sizes that matter, but the proportions of each different nutrient type and how it's set up on your plate. It is also assumed that most bariatric plates will be smaller. So in the diagram above, the bariatric meal plate ideally would be on a much smaller plate vs the average size of a standard dinner plate, hence the portions being different increments.

My version of the bariatric meal plate method is something I call **The Bariatric Breakthrough Meal Plate Method®**. This is the method I use with all my clients and the members in my program. Again, every bariatric RD seems to have their own interpretation of this, and no one is better than the other. It's all just our own takes on how to teach these different proportions and pairing of nutrients. So if you have used something similar before that looks a bit different than the visuals you see here, that's okay. The concepts and reasons for how to use this approach remain the same.

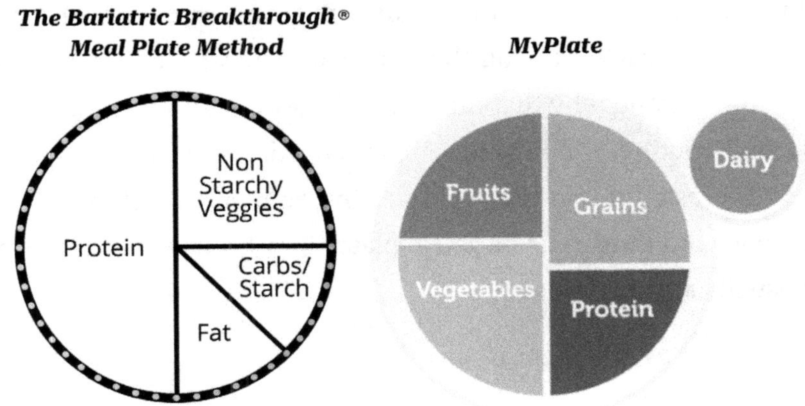

Graphic of the Bariatric Breakthrough Meal Plate Method next to the graphic of the MyPlate graphic, showing how portions vary.

So in regards to the portion suggestions as you progress through your diet, what I also want you to know is that what those portions CONSIST of matters! And I want you to fully understand the WHY behind how to set up your plates after surgery and tackle your nutrition.

Below is an example of how you might progress your meals over time, using the meal plate method and the suggested portions for each diet stage.

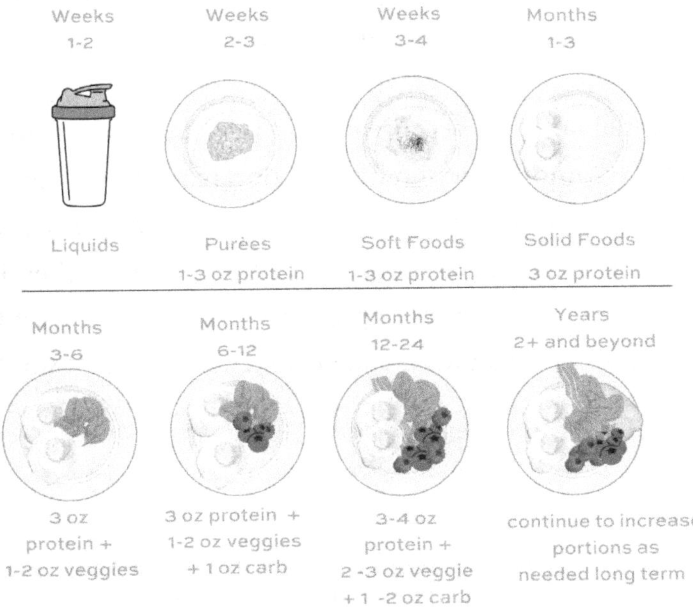

Graphics of bariatric meal plate progression, showing how portion sizes increase and variety expands over time.

Now for the fun part! I'm going to dive into each section of the meal plate and explain and teach it to you the same way I do with all my clients, so you will fully understand why that nutrient is important, how and when to add it back to your routine, and how this approach will serve you long term on your journey! There's a lot that goes into healing your relationship with food, but starting with building your bariatric plates in a healthful and nonrestrictive way is usually a good first step.

Protein

When it comes to post-op nutrition, protein is key. Protein will always take priority over any other nutrient on your plate. The main reason for this is because protein is the most essential nutrient to avoid malnutrition. According to the WHO, malnutrition refers to deficiencies, excesses, or imbalances in a person's intake of energy and/or nutrients.[90] Malnutrition is defined as the lack of proper nutrition, caused by not having enough to eat, not eating enough of the right things, or being unable to use the food that one does eat. And it's a myth that you can't suffer from malnutrition while simultaneously being overweight or obese. Morbidly obese people suffer from malnutrition as well. Malnutrition can lead to very serious and irreversible consequences, including severe nutrient and vitamin and mineral deficiencies.

Protein is the most essential nutrient, because protein is so important in order for your body to function. Almost every bodily function relies on protein. It's used just about everywhere—in muscle, bone, skin, hair, and virtually every other body part or tissue. It makes up the enzymes that power many chemical reactions and the hemoglobin that carries oxygen in your blood. At least ten thousand different proteins make you what you are and keep you that way.[91]

---

[90] WHO, "Malnutrition."

[91] "Protein," "Nutrition Source: What Should I Eat?" section of Harvard T. H. Chan School of Public Health website, accessed on July 14, 2023, https://www.hsph.harvard.edu/nutritionsource/what-should-you-eat/protein.

So in other words, it's REALLY important. It's so important that if you don't give your body enough of it, your body knows to draw from its own protein stores—like your hair, muscles, nails, etc. This is where muscle wasting and hair loss can occur (along with vitamin, mineral, and protein deficiencies).

So how much protein should you be eating to avoid this? Per the ASMBS guidelines, it's suggested that bariatric patients consume at least 60 grams of protein per day. That 60 grams is the absolute minimum. I find that most people tend to do better with closer to 80–90 grams of protein, if they are able to achieve that. Macronutrient needs are individualized, so make sure you are speaking to your clinical bariatric team about what personal protein goal they recommend for you. Many bariatric patients will need to supplement with protein shakes and supplements in order to hit their protein goals, especially early on in their journey. It's okay to rely on shakes.

BUT I do encourage you to do your best to work on eating whole-food sources of protein to work towards hitting your protein goal. The reason it's important for bariatric patients to focus on whole protein sources is so that they can truly learn how to USE their new tool long term. Over time, once you're able to eat more, you will need to rely on protein to keep you fuller and maximize your restriction.

One of the things I see happening often in the bariatric community is patients relying solely on protein shakes to hit their protein goal. What I see happening is they will reach the minimum 60 grams of protein per day by drinking two 30-gram protein shakes and then eating other foods that may not be serving them or filling them up properly. Long term, this can lead to overeating.

In regards to the bariatric meal plate method, I suggest bariatric patients focus on filling at least half of their plates with protein before adding other nutrient types to it. Now, that's not because other food groups are "bad" or because I want you to avoid food groups; it's because protein is so essential to avoiding malnutrition and learning to use your WLS properly that it has to take priority above all else, especially in those first few months. However, there is one caveat to this. I ONLY suggest making half your plate protein if you are getting at least 3 ounces of protein in at a time.

So for example: if you are only able to eat 4 ounces of food maximum in one sitting, I do NOT suggest eating 2 ounces of protein to make it half your overall portion. I like to see everyone eating at least 3 ounces of protein first, before fully implementing the meal plate method.

And there is a very simple reason I suggest at least 3 ounces of whole protein foods on your plate before progressing to other foods: it ensures that you will meet 60 grams per day.

If you only remember one thing from this chapter let it be this:

Every 1 ounce of lean protein = 7 grams of protein (approximately).

Now, let's use some simple math to apply that.

Hypothetically, if you are eating 3 ounces of protein, that is approximately 21 grams of protein per meal. If you focus on three meals per day, that will bring you right up to 63 grams of protein per day (give or take).

Foods that count toward your protein goal: poultry (chicken/turkey), eggs, lean beef, low-fat dairy (low-fat cheese, cottage cheese, yogurt), fish, shellfish, tofu, and edamame.

Some will be able to hit this goal relatively easily. Others may struggle to eat 3 ounces of protein at a time first. That's okay. THIS is when I think it is good to rely on supplements or to have shakes or other high-protein snacks in between meals.

Veggies and Fiber

Once you are consistently able to hit your protein goals by eating at least 3 ounces of protein, the next foods I suggest adding back into your routine are non-starchy veggies.

There are so many options when it comes to adding veggies to your meals, but some examples of non-starchy veggies include the following: broccoli, cauliflower, peppers, cucumber, zucchini, eggplant, spinach, arugula, lettuce, mushrooms, green beans, fennel, tomatoes, snow peas, celery, and okra. I also suggest counting carrots towards your non-starchy veggie goal.

Non-starchy vegetables add dietary fiber to your diet. Dietary fiber is not able to be broken down or digested by the body, so it's often referred to as "roughage" or "bulk." This is SO important for digestion (so if you struggle with constipation post-op, adding veggies and high-fiber fruits can be incredibly helpful).

Dietary fiber recommendations for men: 38 grams

Dietary fiber recommendations for women: 25 grams

It's unlikely that, as a bariatric patient, you will be able to fulfill these daily recommendations through food intake alone, so fiber supplementation can be helpful. There are also other ways, beyond just veggies, to get fiber in. But the reason non-starchy vegetables are particularly beneficial for bariatric patients, even more so than some of the other dietary fiber sources (like fruits and whole grains, which we will get into), is because they take extra long to break down and digest. Early on, in the first year after surgery, you may not be able to tolerate a lot of vegetables, especially raw ones. That's okay, and that's normal. No one is expecting you to be able to add tons of veggies right away. But in terms of maximizing your restriction, like we talked about with the protein, veggies are going to truly help fill your pouch and keep you fuller longer, because your body has to work harder to try and break them down (which it can't do) before it's excreted. Over time, as you are able to eat more and start to feel hungrier again, that protein and veggie combo is the ultimate powerhouse skill to truly use your pouch long term. The other wonderful part about these two nutrients being consumed first, in addition to everything previously mentioned, is that you can add quite a bit of both without significantly adding calories to your routine. While increasing calories is important over time—and your calories SHOULD increase—in terms of making sure you're not unintentionally eating "too much" calorically over time, adding these nutrients to your meals is a great way to get your needs met, stay full, and avoid overeating.

Carbohydrates

Ahhhh yes, everyone's favorite topic. Every time I teach my clients about carbs, I like to preface my lesson by acknowledging that carbs are overwhelming and hard for a lot of us. So if the thought of eating carbohydrates overwhelms you, if you feel guilty or shameful for eating carbs, or you have a troubled relationship with carbs, I just want to take a moment to acknowledge that and to validate anyone who may have an intense emotional response to eating (or not eating) carbohydrates.

There just is so much misinformation about carbohydrates. Society repeatedly tells us they are "bad" and cause weight gain. That's not true. It's not that carbs are "bad"; it's that they are different in structure than other nutrients. Protein and high-fiber veggies keep us fuller and take longer to digest and breakdown, and carbohydrates are much easier to digest. Carbohydrates also tend to be more palatable, depending on the type, which can make them a go-to source for quick energy. For many of us, that quick energy easily translates to a "quick hit" of dopamine in moments of anxiety, stress, or emotions. In addition, carbohydrate consumption can contribute to your body holding on to water, which can also sometimes leave people with the illusion that carbs make them "bloated" or "puffy."

So between restricting them throughout different times of our life, feeling deprived of something our body needs, sometimes feeling bloated after eating them, and not knowing HOW to eat them to make sure they are keeping us full (and not just serving as a quick sugar source), it's no wonder carbs are so feared.

So let's lay out some facts and educational information about carbs. I think if we can zoom out, put aside the emotions, and truly understand the science behind what a carb is, what it does, and how it works, we can help you make more empowered choices around how you choose to eat them after surgery.

First and foremost, carbohydrates are the body's preferred source of energy. When you eat a carbohydrate, regardless of what kind, it is broken down into glucose. Glucose is the sugar in the body that is utilized for energy.

While all carbohydrates are broken down into sugar, not all carbohydrates are the same. There are two different classifications of carbohydrates: simple and complex carbohydrates.

Simple Carbohydrates

I like to think of simple carbohydrates as more "simple in structure." **Simple carbohydrate sources include the following:** white bread, pasta, pastries, bagels, crackers, chips, cookies, rice cakes, cheese puffs, pretzels, etc.

When you think about simple carbohydrates, I want you to think of "snacky foods." NOT "junk food." Let's try and remove that verbiage from our overall food dialogue. Remember, carbs (and foods in general) are not "good" or "bad" but "different."

Simple carbohydrates are often referred to as "slider" foods in our community because, essentially, they "slide" through your pouch or stomach more quickly because there isn't much to them to keep you full. They lack fiber and protein and are in their simplest form already.

I want you to pause for a second. I want you to picture what it feels like to chew a cracker or a Cheeto (cheese puff). Now I want you to picture eating a bite of chicken. Picture what it feels like to chew it and even swallow it.

My guess is when you envision yourself chewing those different foods, they feel very different. That's because they ARE very different, primarily in how they are digested and in what they actually DO in the body.

Digestion begins as soon as you start chewing for carbohydrates. I'm not sure if you know this, but chewing is considered a mechanical process of digestion. As you chew, your mouth produces saliva. Saliva has different bacteria and enzymes that aid in the chemical digestion.

Interestingly enough, we have an enzyme in our saliva that is called **amylase**. Amylase breaks down carbohydrates into sugar as soon as you start chewing. Ever notice how when you eat a Cheeto, it almost disappears or disintegrates as you are chewing it? It's almost like there is nothing left to it by the time you swallow, whereas protein does not start to denature and digest until it hits your stomach acid. In your stomach, and throughout your small intestine, there is an enzyme called **pepsin**, which is an enzyme that breaks down protein. So it makes sense why protein keeps you fuller longer.

So if you've ever reached for a simple carbohydrate or "snacky" food and wondered, *"How in the world can I eat SO much of this still after surgery*?" You're not alone, my friend. It's not you, and your pouch isn't broken. There is a reason those types of carbohydrates are so easily digested. They don't contain nutrients or fiber. Your body just very readily breaks down the sugar.

When we eat simple carbohydrates alone (meaning not paired with any other nutrient), not only does it not keep us as full, but we tend to feel even hungrier. And yes, as you might have guessed, there is another scientific reason for this.

As you break down your food into glucose, that glucose is released into the bloodstream. When glucose enters the bloodstream, your pancreas produces and releases insulin. By definition, insulin is a

> peptide hormone secreted by the β cells of the pancreatic islets of Langerhans that maintains normal blood glucose levels by facilitating cellular glucose uptake; regulating carbohydrate, lipid, and protein metabolism; and promoting cell division and growth through its mitogenic effects.[92]

But more simply put, insulin is the hormone that allows your cells to use that glucose in your bloodstream for energy.

When you eat a simple carbohydrate, it not only physically does not keep you very full, it also creates a large increase in blood sugar. What happens (very simply put) is this: you have a rush of blood sugar, insulin is quickly released to bring it back down, and then your blood sugar gets low very quickly. Have you ever had a really high-carbohydrate breakfast (like a donut or pastry) or had a very large sugar-sweetened beverage (like a milkshake) and, despite it being higher in calories, about an hour later, you feel ravenously hungry or even shaky? That's because having that simple carbohydrate spikes your blood sugar quickly, and then it plummets quickly too.

Unless you are an athlete and are training for some type of intense physical goal, having very quick-and-simple carbohydrate sources usually isn't going to be to your benefit. They are foods you are more likely to overeat, as they won't keep you very full and will leave you feeling hungrier throughout the day. And because of that quick sugar rush, they tend to be the "dopamine hit" or "sugar fix" a lot of us crave and want. So to top it off, they are also foods you are more likely to lean on emotionally.

In no way am I suggesting you shouldn't eat simple carbs; I think that is wild-

[92] Gisela Wilcox, "Insulin and Insulin Resistance," Clinical Biochemist Reviews 26, no. 2 (May 2005): 19–39, https://www.ncbi.nlm.nih.gov/pmc/articles/PMC1204764/.

ly unrealistic and honestly not helpful. Because again, it's not that they are bad. Your body just digests them and responds to them differently. This is WHY, when you start to add carbs back into your diet, I suggest eating them in smaller quantities or proportions than the protein and veggies, and it is also why I always suggest pairing them with other nutrients on your plate. If you eat a simple carb in addition to a protein and veggies source, you are less likely to experience the negative effects of unintentionally over eating them.

Complex Carbohydrates

Once you are able to get your protein needs met and add veggies to your diet regularly and you still have room for more food or are still finding yourself hungry or dissatisfied, that's when I suggest adding carbs into your routine. And I always suggest starting with a complex carb, if possible, as opposed to a simple carbohydrate.

I like to think of complex carbohydrates as more "complicated in structure." **Complex carbohydrate sources include the following foods:** whole grain breads/whole-wheat products, oatmeal, brown rice/brown rice products, quinoa, beans, legumes, and fruits.

These carbohydrates are digested the exact same way as simple carbohydrates. HOWEVER, these carbs contain fiber. They also contain lots of other nutrients and even water, if we are looking at the content of fruit. This is going to ultimately take up more stomach space and have the same bulking effect that veggies have. These carbohydrates take longer to digest, making the release of sugar to the bloodstream, as well as the uptake of glucose into the cells with insulin, slower. Because this process is slower, they likely will keep you fuller longer and also help maximize your restriction.

Adding Carbs Back In

For a lot of bariatric patients, it can feel really intimidating to add carbs back into your routine. A lot of people are fearful of adding them in, because they worry it will stop or stall their weight loss.

Carbohydrates do hold on to water, so it's not unusual to notice a bit of water retention or fluctuations on the scale when first introducing carbs back in. This is also why if you cut carbs OUT, a lot of people usually will notice a loss on the scale. But just know, that loss is usually water, and it's not sustainable to keep carbs out of your body, especially long term.

It's all about how you eat them. Try to stick with the rule of thumb and pair them with your protein and another fiber source. I always want your goals coming from a place of abundance, not scarcity. So rather than focusing on what you *won't* eat, focus on what you can *add* to your meals or snack plates to make them *more* nutritious, *more* satisfying, and *more* filling. And make sure you are following your surgery center's post-op diet. If they don't want you adding certain foods back in right away, don't. While you likely won't be adding many carbs initially, with time, they will likely become a part of your life again. And when they do, I hope this helps you feel more prepared for how to incorporate them into your routine.

Fat

Myth: fat makes you fat. I am happy to report back: it does not. Fat is an essential nutrient for the body, just like the others. The one thing to keep in mind is fat is more calorically dense than the other nutrients.

Macronutrient	Calories per gram
Protein	4 calories/gram
Carbohydrate	4 calories/gram
Fat	9 calories/gram

The calories for fat are more than double that per gram of protein and carb, which means smaller portions add up more calories. I think the most disappointing moment of my life was when I actually measured out what a true serving size of peanut butter is. Okay, that might be dramatic, but it's pretty sad when you see what a true tablespoon of peanut butter weighed out on the food scale actually looks like. That doesn't mean I want you obsessing over every gram of peanut butter or salad dressing; I just want you to be aware and mindful of the fact that high-fat foods are going to contribute a lot more calories to your overall intake—which, similar to simple carbs, makes them easy to overeat at times, depending on the source.

Foods that count as a fat source include the following: butter/nut butters, seeds, nuts, dressings, full fat dairy and cheese, avocado, oils, dips, spreads, etc.

I don't love the term "healthy fat sources." I think it reinforces the "good and bad" food mentality that we are trying to break free of. Scientifically speaking, at the end of the day, a fat source is a fat source. But it is true that not all fat sources are created equal. For example, foods high in oil or fried foods will add up in calories much more quickly than say an avocado, which is a whole-food source of fat that is also naturally higher in fiber. Not to mention, fried foods are usually consumed in conjunction with breading or simple carbohydrates that also won't keep you particularly full. And a lot of bariatric patients find that foods high in fats can upset their stomachs or make them sick.

When looking at the bariatric meal plate method, it's a little challenging to visually show how to incorporate it into the plate. One of the reasons for this is fat sources tend to naturally make their way to your plate by way of meat, dairy, and/or different flavors or cooking agents. So when it comes to adding food to your plate "in order" (as I teach, leading with protein, then veggies, then carbs), fat is the one caveat. I don't expect you to "wait" to add fat back in. It's going to be there. The bigger takeaway when looking at it visually is the portion size/its proportion to the other nutrients. For most people, having an ounce or 1 to 2 tablespoons of fat on their plate is sufficient and makes sense. The reason fat is so important is because fat brings "satiety" to our diet. Fat has what's called a "mouth feel." Picture eating homemade macaroni and cheese or homemade cornbread with butter. It leaves almost a coating or film in your mouth that gives you that "comfort" food sensation. It is ultimately what allows you to feel satisfied when you eat, or at least increase your level of satisfaction.

Have you ever done a really low-fat diet before? I can remember back in my Weight Watchers era, in an attempt to keep my points as low as possible, I would choose foods that were either zero points or very low points, which ultimately meant eating very low-fat meals.

One of those meals was often salad with fat-free dressing and chicken with no cheese, no nuts, no croutons, and avocado. I mean . . . is there anything less satisfying or less palatable? Eating meals like this often leads to overeating later, or feeling like you "just need something else" after your meal, even if you are full.

This goes back to my "abundance" versus "scarcity" mentality. Rather than trying to keep your meals as low calorie or low-fat as possible for the sake of keeping your intakes low and "healthy," I would much rather you add a serving of fat to your meal. Make it MORE satisfying. If you make that salad (lettuce/veggies with chicken and fat-free or low-fat dressing), I would either suggest swapping out the dressing for one a little higher in fat for satisfaction and fullness OR adding some cheese or avocado. That would make it SO much tastier, so much more satisfying, and a more fulfilling meal overall.

Not to mention, fat is so important for proper nutrient absorption. Vitamins A, D, E, and K are fat soluble, so they need fat in order to be absorbed. If your diet is very low in fat, it's going to be even harder to properly absorb your vitamins.

The Goal: To Get Back to a Normal, Balanced Diet

The big picture here is it's important to feed and nourish your body. Just because you had weight loss surgery doesn't mean you should be eating infant-sized portions forever. The whole point is to get back to a normal, healthful, sustainable food routine in which all foods fit.

It's also important for bariatric patients to focus on building meals as much as possible. The more you can focus on creating high-protein plates and building them out with other nutrients over time, the better you will be able to utilize your tool (aka, your bariatric stomach) and the fuller you will feel.

I tell my clients this: all foods fit, just not all the time. There is a process. You start off with very small and restricted portions, but over time, it's so essential that you add foods back in. It's unrealistic to expect to eat teeny-tiny portions of protein only for the rest of your life. You are a living human being who needs energy. And I really believe the first step to healing your relationship with food is to understand how it works and why we need the nutrients we need in the order in which we need them.

And above all else, I want you to be realistic with your food and weight loss expectations.

Bite-Sized Recap

- Nutrition is what you will eat, not what you won't eat.
- The goal after weight loss surgery is not to eat as little as possible for as long as possible. The goal is to nourish your body, feed it, and give it all the nutrients it needs to thrive and function.
- Everyone's portions are going to look different after weight loss surgery.
- The diet progression comes with time. Over time, you will be able to eat more food.
- Most bariatric patients benefit from eating protein first, then non-starchy veggies, and eventually high-fiber carbohydrates and fat for flavor.
- All foods fit, just not all the time.
- There is a process. You start off with very small and restricted portions, but over time, it's essential that you add foods back in. It's unrealistic to expect to only eat teeny-tiny portions of protein for the rest of your life.

For journal prompts and resources related to this chapter be sure to head to www.thesleeveddietitian.com/easy.

Chapter 8
Let's Be Realistic

re·al·is·tic
/rēəlistik/
adjective
1. having or showing a sensible and practical idea of what can be achieved or expected
"Restrictive diets are short-term fixes, so you've got to be realistic."
2. representing familiar things in a way that is accurate or true to life
"A realistic routine you can stick with is ideal."

Let's Be Real

One of the beauties of being both a dietitian and bariatric patient is that I've been able to see what works "on paper" versus what *actually* works.

Unfortunately, a lot of bariatric patients have unrealistic expectations when it comes to what they will and won't eat, how much they will eat, and how much weight they are going to lose and keep off after surgery. And honestly? When I see people come to me with unrealistic expectations, I don't fault them. If anything, I fault those who did not properly educate or prepare them.

It's frustrating when someone comes to me with unrealistic expectations put upon them by their surgical centers. So often, I see people with post-op diets that state things like:

"No carbohydrates for life."

"No snacks after surgery."

"No more than 1,000 calories per day for life."

So with rules like these, what happens? Well, what happens is people aren't able to follow them for obvious reasons, like we just talked about. We need carbs. We need to have snacks sometimes. And I don't know any human over the age of two who should be eating 1,000 calories per day for life.

And when people aren't able to follow these rules, they immediately think or assume they are failing. But the goals laid in front of them were never attainable to begin with.

The truth is, you will be able to eat more. You should be able to eat more. And realistically, you need to figure out how to have a routine you can stick with long term, as time goes on and your goals (and your weight) shifts and changes. Along with pigeonholing yourself with such strict expectations, it's also detrimental when you don't prepare for the fact that your weight loss goals need to be realistic, just as much as your food goals need to be.

In order to set ourselves up for success, we need to be realistic. And the first step to being realistic is to throw out the idea of perfection. No one is perfect. Perfect on this journey doesn't even exist. Sure, you need to follow your post-op diet as closely as possible, but that post-op diet is short-lived. After the strict diet phase ends, you must rely on the habits that will support you long term. No one should be trying to eat the way they did at two months post-op for the rest of their lives. Perfection always sets us up for disappointment. Rather than focusing on being perfect, I'd rather you make the adjustments you need to in order to be consistent.

I want you to not only understand nutrition and habits to set yourself up for success, but I want you to know how to apply them in a way that works for you and helps you stay consistent long term. Below are some things that I see bariatric patients either getting overwhelmed by or consumed with, which leads them into all-or-nothing thinking. As an alternative, I'm going to clarify any myths or confusion and help you understand some practical ways you can apply these skills and habits to your routine realistically.

Calorie Awareness, Not Obsession

As a bariatric dietitian I get asked all the time about calories and macros. Bariatric patients are always concerned about how many calories they should be eating. So I'm going to break it down for you and give you my thoughts.

What is a Calorie?

A calorie is a unit of energy. All food is made up of calories in order to provide our bodies with the energy needed to function. Every part of our body (our cells, brains, muscles, etc.) requires energy to live. According to an article in the *Journal of Nutrition*, "History of the Calorie in Nutrition," in 1863, a calorie was defined "as the amount of heat needed to raise the temperature of 1 kilogram of water from 0 to 1 degree Celsius."[93] But in more simple terms, a calorie is a unit of energy. And in order to lose weight, you need to be in a calorie deficit. I'm sure many of you have heard the term "calories in versus calories out." A calorie deficit occurs when we burn or expend more than we consume.

What is a Macro?

The term "macro" refers to macronutrients. There are three macronutrients: protein, carbohydrates, and fats. Each of these three things provides us with different amounts of calories, like we discussed in the previous chapter.

When people say they are counting their macros, what they are doing is counting where their calories are coming from. So rather than just counting overall calories, they aim to hit certain macronutrient goals that will make up their

[93] James L. Hargrove, "History of the Calorie in Nutrition," *Journal of Nutrition* 136, no. 12 (December 2006): 2957–2961, https://jn.nutrition.org/article/S0022-3166(22)08554-6/fulltext.

overall calories and are tracking where their calories are coming from.

Should You Be Counting Calories and Macros?

Personally, I think counting macros is incredibly overwhelming and unnecessary. The only macronutrient I recommend counting or focusing on is protein. Aim to hit a minimum of 60 grams of protein per day OR the individualized goal set for you by your bariatric team.

However, if you genuinely enjoy macro counting or are using macros to hit a certain fitness goal, as long as it doesn't create disordered thoughts or habits, I think it can be okay for certain individuals. But it definitely isn't an approach that works for everyone, or even the majority.

Some people really enjoy tracking their food (both calories and macros), and to them I say, that's great! If you are someone who genuinely enjoys tracking your food, and it helps keep you accountable, then I think tracking can be a really great tool.

There are many people, though, who don't do well with tracking their food intake long term. For some, what starts off as "accountability" can quickly lead to "obsession" or even disordered eating and thinking.

One of the number one questions I get asked is this: *"Jamie, how many calories should I be eating?"* Or *"I'm [insert how many months or years post-op]; how many calories should I be eating at this stage?"*

There are a lot of misconceptions around calorie intake and needs. When I get asked these questions, my response is always the same: *"Unfortunately, I can' tell you that. Not because I don't want to help you, but because there genuinely isn't a right answer."*

Everyone's calorie and macro needs are completely individualized. In order to calculate your calories and macros, you need to factor in your age, gender, height, weight, exercise/energy expenditure, and your personal eating habits and goals. And the only person who should be calculating this for you is a registered dietitian who knows and works with you individually. So if you message someone on social media and say, "How many calories should I be eating?" and the person actually gives you a number, RUN. They don't know what they are doing. And if you ask someone at your surgical center, and they give you a generic answer like "1,000 calories" or "1,200 calories" without factoring in everything I mentioned above, fire them and go find a new provider.

One of the rebuttals I hear often when I tell people that their RD is the only person who should be giving them individual calorie and macro goals is this: "But, Jamie, I asked her, and she wouldn't give me one." And to be honest, when I hear this, it's like music to my ears. If your surgery center will not give you customized calorie goals or macro "limits," it tells me you have a really great surgical center that cares about your long-term success. Let me explain.

When I was first having my weight loss surgery, I remember being SO frustrated with my dietitian, because she wouldn't give me a calorie goal or a carb limit, despite my repeated asking. Now, could I have just calculated my needs myself, since I am a dietitian? Sure, I could have. But I wanted the structure. I wanted the rules. I felt like if she could give me stricter rules to follow, I could prove to everyone that I was going to be the most "perfect" bariatric patient they ever saw and I would know exactly what to do to hit all my goals.

Looking back, had she given me those "rules," I would have been at a huge disadvantage. If strict calorie and macro counting worked, none of us would have needed surgery to begin with. Rather than using an outside tool (tracking), my dietitian really encouraged me to start to listen to and trust my body and use the new internal tool I had.

I think having a general awareness surrounding calories and macros is important. And it's true, you need to be in a calorie deficit in order to lose weight.

The thing is, though, if you had surgery and are utilizing the meal plate method and focusing on protein first and high-fiber options, it's very unlikely you won't be in a calorie deficit.

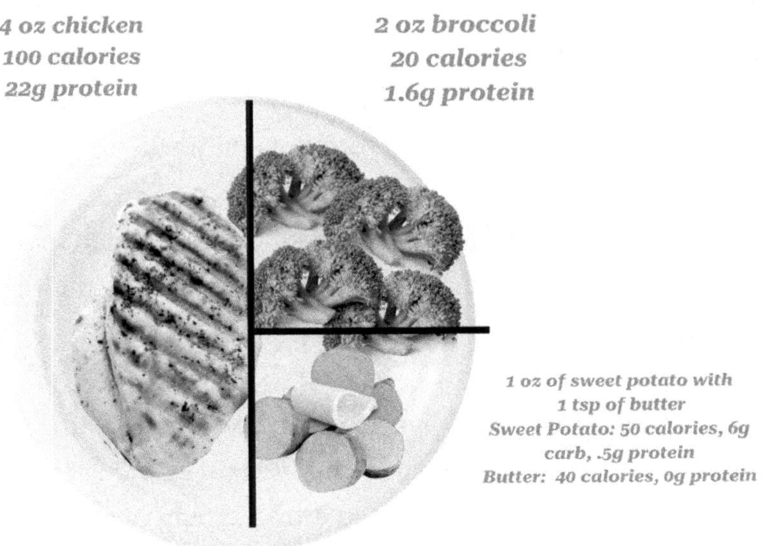

Graphic of a plate showing ½ of the plate containing chicken, ¼ of the plate containing broccoli, and ¼ of the plate divided equally between sweet potato and butter.

If you are utilizing this strategy, along with listening to your body and making sure you are eating when you're hungry and stopping when you're full, it's very unlikely you will not be in a calorie deficit—at least in those first couple of years.

Obsessing about every single calorie or carb you put into your body isn't going to benefit you. All it's going to do, for most people, is cause another unhealthy relationship with food and fear around calories and different nutrients.

Many people come to me and say, "Oh my God, Jamie, my calories are so much higher than I think they should be. What should I do?" What's interesting is I see this a lot with people in their first year post-op. What often happens is they get accustomed to seeing 500–800 calories or so per day in those first few weeks or months, and then they are suddenly in a 1,000–1,500 calorie range. I get why this is alarming; I really do. It's easy to judge yourself and fear you're eating too much. But interestingly enough, so many of these people are panicking just from seeing that number, not taking a moment to zoom out and recognize they are still losing weight and (usually) feeling more energized. I'm a big believer in the motto "don't fix what isn't broken." Just because you are eating more doesn't mean you aren't on the right track.

Again, eating isn't bad. You need to eat, and your calories should increase. And if you are still losing weight, even if it's more slowly, then you can rest assured you are in a calorie deficit.

My best piece of advice is to stop hyperfocusing on these arbitrary numbers just because it's what you "think" you should be eating. And at the end of the day, counting your calories and macros in a tracker app is just a really good estimation of what your body is keeping track of anyways. Unless you are perfectly weighing every gram of food and every bite you ever take, your calorie count isn't accurate anyway. But your body is a natural food diary. It takes account of everything accurately, regardless of what you have written on paper. And I don't know about you, but nothing sounds worse to me than weighing out every gram of food and perfectly tracking it for the rest of my life. The thought actually makes me dizzy.

That's no way to live. I want you to learn really great habits you can stick with, so you can go out into the world and actually LIVE. I want you to feel confident traveling, going to picnics and parties, and spending time with those you love without being afraid of every single calorie and macro.

Calorie awareness is important. Knowing that highly refined carbohydrates and high-fat foods will add up in terms of calories is important. But this is where I want you to take this education and apply it in real life. Be mindful of your portions. Create boundaries for yourself and your habits. Use that meal plate method. And listen to your body.

It's what you do most of the time, not some of the time, that matters most. So if most of the time you are choosing really nutritious high-protein options, it's okay if some of the time your plates don't look "perfect." Perfect never existed anyway.

Label Reading

I see a lot of people getting really overwhelmed with and consumed by label reading too. I think this one goes hand in hand with the calorie obsession. A lot of people look at a food label, see that the calories are higher than they think they "should" be, and put the item back. Or sometimes, they look at the "wrong" pieces of the label.

Breaking Down the Nutrition Label

If looking at all of this is overwhelming, that's okay; I'm going to break it down even further.

Personally, I don't think it's necessary to look at the percent daily values, the saturated/trans fat, or the cholesterol—unless, of course, you've been instructed to do so by your medical team. If you struggle with high blood pressure, you may also want to take note of the sodium, but for the majority of the bariatric population, having some extra sodium to get in more electrolytes can actually be helpful.

I think the most important things to look at on the nutrition label are the serving size, the total fat, the carb content, and the protein.

Now, this is where I want to help you get out of that all-or-nothing perfectionist mentality—there isn't any one number you should be looking for. There isn't any one number on any one section of this label that is going to tell you if the food is "good" or "bad."

1 This tells you how many servings are in the container. In this example, there are 8 servings of milk in the container.

2 This tells you the size of ONE serving. In this case ONE serving is ONE cup. This means there are 110 Calories in ONE cup.

3 This tells you how many Calories are in each serving. In this example, there are 110 Calories in every 1-Cup serving.

4 This tells you how much Fat is in each serving. In this example, there are 2.5g of fat in every 1-Cup serving. Out of the 2.5g of Fat, 1.5g is Saturated fat.

5 The Carbohydrate section tells you how many total grams of carbs are in ONE serving. It also tells you how many grams are from fiber, added sugars, and total sugars in each serving.

6 This tells you how much Protein is in each serving. In this example, there are 8g of Protein in every 1-Cup serving.

Nutrition Facts

1 8 servings per container	
2 **Serving size**	**1 Cup (240 mL)**
Amount per serving	
3 **Calories**	**110**
	7 **% Daily Value***
4 **Total Fat** 2.5g	**3%**
Saturated Fat 1.5g	**8%**
Trans Fat 0g	
Cholesterol 15mg	**5%**
Sodium 130mg	**6%**
5 **Total Carbohydrate** 12g	**4%**
Dietary Fiber 0g	**0%**
Total Sugars 12g	
Includes 0g Added Sugars	**0%**
6 **Protein** 8g	**16%**
Vitamin D 2.5mcg	15%
Calcium 310mg	25%
Iron 0.1mg	0%
Potassium 400mg	8%
Vitamin A 150mcg	15%

*The % Daily Value tells you how much a nutrient in a serving of food contributes to a daily diet. 2,000 calories a day is used for general nutrition advice.

This label is from **1% Milk**

7 The % Daily Value (on the right hand side of every row) shows you how much of a nutrient is in one serving, based on a 2,000 Calorie diet. These percentages may not apply to you.

Image of a nutrition label showing the nutritional breakdown of a 8oz cup of 1% milk.

Serving Sizes

The serving size is really important. Without it, there is no frame of reference. The serving size determines all the numbers to follow. It's important to realize that there can be multiple serving sizes in a container or a package.

Total Fat

When you look at the total fat, there isn't any one number to cap yourself at. However, since you already know that fat is more calorically dense, just know that if the total fat is a larger number, the calories of that item will be higher too. If foods high in fat cause you to feel sick, you definitely want to be aware of highly fattening items. If you do choose a food with a high-fat content, just work it into your whole day or whole routine and be mindful of portions.

Total Protein

The higher the protein, the better! Again, there isn't any one protein number to look for, but generally speaking, I suggest looking for products that have more protein than carbs or fat—OR, at the very least, have the equivalent amount of protein to carbs/fat.

Carbohydrates

Looking at the carbs on the nutrition label is easily the most overwhelming part to interpret. I'm going to walk you through each piece of this.

Breaking Down the Nutrition Label: Carbohydrates

Total Carbohydrates	This is the total amount of carbs in the item. It is made up of fiber and sugar. Every 15 grams of carbs equals 1 carb serving. When following the meal plate method, I suggest 1–2 carb servings after your protein needs are met.
Dietary Fiber	The higher the fiber, the better! Fiber helps keep us fuller longer. Fiber isn't digestible, so it takes our body longer to try and break down the food, which is why we stay full. And it helps with staying regular.
Total Sugar	Sugar doesn't automatically mean "bad." But we do want to be mindful of it. Something with lots of fruit might have a higher total sugar content, but this is a little different than added sugar.
Added Sugar	We want to try and choose foods that are lower in added sugar. Higher added-sugar foods are more likely to be slider foods or foods that don't keep us as full.

When it comes to looking at the carbohydrates on a label, my suggestion is this: depending on if it's a meal or a snack option, try and keep your total carbohydrate serving to about 15–30 grams (1–2 carb servings). Unless, of course, you are trying to increase your carbs, perhaps for training purposes. Then, look at the fiber and the added sugar content in comparison to the overall carbohydrate amount. I usually suggest trying to choose something that has more fiber and less sugar. If you notice that the label has very little or no fiber and a lot of added sugar, then it might be a "slider food." But by now, you're a pro at this! So you know that even if it is a simple carbohydrate or slider food, it can still work into your routine, as long as you are pairing it with other nutrients on your plate.

Net Carbs

Whenever I teach people about carbs, I always get asked about net carbs. Net carbs is primarily a marketing term. A lot of people will count net carbs when following a low-carb or "keto" diet. However, THIS is where a lot of people get caught up in the marketing scheme. Even low-net-carb products still have carbohydrates.

total carb
- dietary fiber
- sugar alcohols

---

net carbs

"Net carbs" does not mean "no carbs," and it certainly doesn't mean "no calories." The term "net carbs" is not regulated by the FDA. Food companies and brands essentially adopted this term in order to be able to market their products as "lower carb."

The reason for this, as you've learned, is dietary fiber and sugar alcohols/sugar substitutes don't provide our bodies with calories or energy. So the thought process is to deduct these things from the carb count on the nutrition label, since they don't technically "count."

While I love the logic there, that isn't quite how this works out. During manufacturing, many of the "low-carb" products you see that are labeled as "keto" or "low-carb" are fortified with highly processed forms of fiber, usually in the form of IMO syrup, which can still raise blood glucose levels. IMO syrup is not "bad" or dangerous by any means, but it does typically contribute about 3 calories per gram.

It's not that having low-carb products is "bad." I think these types of foods, such as protein bars, low-carb tortillas, and low-carb/low-sugar "dessert" options, can fit nicely into your routine; and oftentimes, these food choices are lower in added sugar and higher in protein, which is wonderful. But the point is, it's silly to think that adding fiber syrup to a product that naturally has carbs will somehow negate or cancel out what's already there. It's kind of like if you were to eat a cookie and sprinkle Benefiber or MiraLAX on top—it doesn't mean the carbs or calories from the cookies magically disappear! (Although, it's a nice thought.)

People who count net carbs tend to consume more carbohydrates and calories over the course of the day than those who simply focus on balanced meals and snacks. This is often why when people follow a keto diet but are eating lots of "diet products" that are "low-carb," they don't see the weight loss they expect. And for the record, no, I don't suggest following a keto diet. The whole reason we had surgery was to get out of that fad-diet mentality. So let's stop falling for diet-culture terms and gimmicks. Instead, let's apply real nutrition knowledge and skills to your choices.

If you are consuming carbohydrates in your diet, I want you to fully know and understand all this. I see so many bariatric patients saying, "Oh, I don't eat carbs," as they promote a Built Bar or Dive Bar (popular protein bars) on their social media page. And I'm throwing absolutely no shade at either of those brands, but the average Built Bar has approximately 18 grams of carbs, and the average Dive Bar has approximately 25–30 grams of carbs.

You know what has less carbs than your protein bars? A thin slice of whole-wheat bread (about 13 grams of carbs) or a clementine (about 7 grams of carbs) Heck, half of a bagel is 27 grams of carbs. I don't know about you, but if I'm adding carbs to my plate, I want to actually ENJOY them and acknowledge that I'm eating them. And I want you to start doing that too. Because remember, carbs aren't bad. And neither is your protein bar. But I want your logic behind what you are choosing to actually make sense! Don't choose the protein bar because it's "low in carbs." Choose it because you want it and it helps you hit your goal for the day, but also acknowledge that having a thin slice of bread with an egg will get the job done too.

Meal Planning

Meal planning and meal prepping tend to give people a lot of anxiety. But you want to know a secret? There's no "right" or "wrong" way to meal prep. I think it's also important to recognize that not everyone has the same abilities when it comes to meal planning and prepping. Especially for those who are neurodivergent or who have disabilities or physical limitations, finding quick meal planning and prepping hacks (such as having ready-made foods ordered) is necessary for so many.

When I think about meal prepping, the first thing that comes to mind is slaving away in the kitchen for an entire Sunday, perfectly portioning and weighing everything I'm going to eat for the whole week. I usually envision one of my favorite fitness influencers, with her perfectly lined-up glass containers and her food scale, making sure every bite is accounted for and tracked for the upcoming week.

Now, just like with calorie or macro counting, if that works for you and you genuinely enjoy it, all the power to you. Don't fix what isn't broken. But if the thought of having to do that makes you immediately just want to order takeout, then I'm with you.

Meal prep doesn't have to be "perfect." And I just don't think it's realistic or sustainable to feel the need to always plan everything to a T. As humans, we want and need variety. Sometimes you aren't in the mood to eat certain things. I don't want you to feel like you need to pigeonhole yourself into eating some perfectly prepped meal plan every week. That doesn't leave room for any flexibility and, therefore, likely won't be a realistic habit to keep up with. It also doesn't help you learn to trust yourself with your day-to-day decision-making or build confidence in listening to your body.

However, that's not to say that planning ahead isn't important. As humans, not even just bariatric patients, it's important we have some kind of game plan for how we are going to feed ourselves each week. But that doesn't mean you have to have a rigid meal plan to follow all the time. If meal plans alone worked, none of us would have struggled with our weight.

If you've been following my own WLS journey on Instagram, you already know that I am a self-proclaimed "lazy meal prepper." I say this proudly, actually. Why make it harder for myself than it has to be?

My motto is work smarter, not harder. This journey is hard enough; let's not further complicate it by trying to preplan and pre-track everything that goes into your mouth. And for the record, that just isn't necessary, especially if you don't enjoy it.

Meal prep can and SHOULD be simple. One of the things I always hear from my clients is "Ugh, I just don't want to think about food anymore!" And what they mean by that is that they don't want to spend every waking moment obsessing about what they will or will not eat every day.

You may have heard the saying "Plan ahead or plan to fail." Will you automatically fail if you aren't planning ahead? No, not necessarily. Again, there are so many nuances in nutrition and lifestyle habits. The key is learning which habits suit you, your goals, and your lifestyle best.

More often than not, having food prepared ahead of time can really help us feel in control of our food choices. It can help minimize obsessing over what to choose and can help us avoid grazing, snacking, or running out for fast food. I'm excited to share with you how to do this in a quick and EASY way.

Meal prepping should be a part of your routine. If the term "meal prep" alone stresses you out, just think of it as meal planning.

By preplanning your meals and getting a good idea of what you will eat throughout the week, you will

- Feel more in control of your routine;
- Feel more confident building your meal plates and staying on track;
- Feel empowered to make choices that align with your goals all week long;
- Minimize stress, snacking, grazing, and mindlessly eating food.

Meal prepping should work with your routine. There is no one right way to go about it. Some people like to batch cook all their food to have ready to go, while others like to cook food every night as they move along.

Personally, my evenings are crunched for time, so I like to cook a couple of big batches of food to keep on hand to mix and match all week long. This is the approach I'm going to share with you, and hopefully you can take what you need from these tips.

My Meal Planning Strategy

STEP 1: DECIDE

You first need to decide what it is you would like to plan on having available to you for the week. Set aside some time either at the beginning or at the end of the week to think about what types of food you would like to prepare for the week, keeping in mind the bariatric meal plate method.

Tips:

- Take a look at your week's schedule.
- Pick one day out of the week to plan out your meals. I like to suggest taking 20–30 minutes to write everything out and prepare a grocery list.
- Think about the foods you LIKE to eat. Prepping chicken and broccoli every night gets OLD, so think about the foods you feel good about eating.

Avoid:

- Choosing overly complicated meals and recipes.
- Trying to eat something different for every meal/snack. Some variety is good, but too much can be overwhelming.

The "Choose 3 Rule":
I'm not usually one for "rules." BUT this one "rule" can save you a LOT of frustration, time, and guesswork. It's what I call the "Choose 3 Rule."

I really encourage you to choose three of each food type (protein, veggie, and carb) to prepare and have ready to go in the fridge. This way, you can mix and match which foods you pair together all week long to create variety, all while using the same ingredients and foods. This can save you time, minimize waste, and help you cut down on the cost of groceries.

Example of the "Choose 3 Rule"

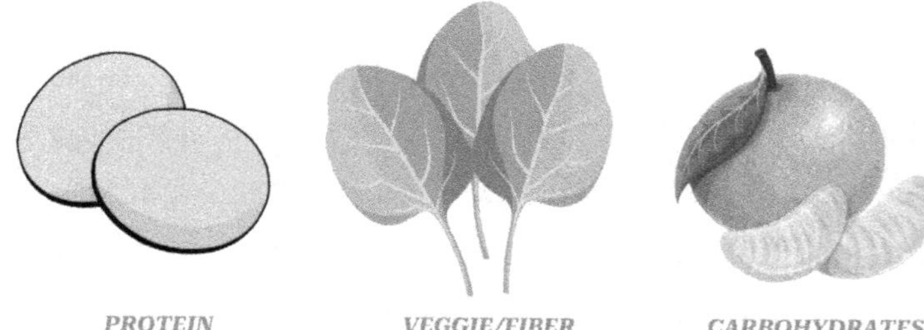

Graphic of eggs, spinach, and a clementine.

Protein	Veggie/Fiber	Carbohydrate
Rotisserie chicken	Prewashed baby spinach	Clementines
Eggs	Bell peppers	Whole-wheat tortilla
Grilled salmon	Grilled zucchini	Roasted sweet potato

**Notice how some of these options require ZERO prep work? Remember, think smarter, not harder!*

STEP 2: PREPARE

Some items you won't have to prepare. (In the example above, the chicken, spinach, clementines, and tortillas require no prep work.)

I'm a firm believer that meal prep should not take that long. If you are spending more than an hour per week meal prepping, it's likely you are over complicating things.

Tips:

- Set time in your week to prepare your meals.
- You may need to also set aside time to either go to the grocery store or place a grocery order to make sure you are ready to prepare your food.
- Pick a day that works for you to purchase food and prepare it. (The days you purchase and prepare can be different days!) Just hold yourself accountable to whatever you choose.
- Pick a day to prepare your food that works for you. If you KNOW Sundays are busy with family activities, then maybe choose a day that is less hectic, as long as it fits into your routine.
- MULTITASK! Cut your fruit while your eggs boil, your chicken cooks in the Instant Pot, and your veggies roast in the oven. Do it all at once! Trust me, you will cut down on prep time.
- You don't have to put things into perfectly portioned containers. Throwing all your chicken into one big container to grab and go or portion later is just fine.
- You can also partially prepare things. For example, maybe you wash and chop up some veggies you plan on stir-frying later in the week. Perhaps doing just that one piece ahead of time will cut down on prep.

STEP 3: MIX & MATCH

The goal is to take everything you have planned and prepared and mix and match the various ingredients and prepped items to create multiple different dishes and meals throughout the week. You can use different sauces (such as sugar-free BBQ, teriyaki, honey mustard, etc.) to add fat and flavor to these meals and variety in taste. For example, with different flavoring, you can change the taste of the chicken or the salmon all week long.

This is where mixing and matching the "Choose 3 Rule" really comes into play.

Again, the goal is to be realistic.

Some weeks you may want to plan out more elaborate meals, but sometimes, keeping it simple is best.

With the examples above, you likely will also want to think about having additional staples in the house to help create variety with the things you've created. Having extra condiments, as well as staples like shredded cheese or avocado, on hand can be helpful. The reason I didn't include the "fats" to prepare is because, as I mentioned earlier, those typically will find their way to our plate by adding flavor.

The "Choose 3 Rule" can be really great for a busy lifestyle. There are so many ways you can use it! This was just ONE way to do it. It all depends on you, your family, the foods you enjoy, and what will be most satisfying.

Remember, your meal prep is a way to keep you on track all week. But please also allow yourself flexibility.

Always listen to your body. Eat when you are hungry and choose foods that sound good to you. Give yourself permission to choose in the moment, all while having the peace of mind of knowing you have a fridge full of options to make a quick bariatric plate on the fly!

Realistic Weight Expectations

Along with being realistic with your food expectations, being realistic with weight expectations is SO important. Weight loss is not linear. I know in our heads we expect that the scale will just keep constantly moving down until we hit our "goal," but the truth is, that's not how weight loss works.

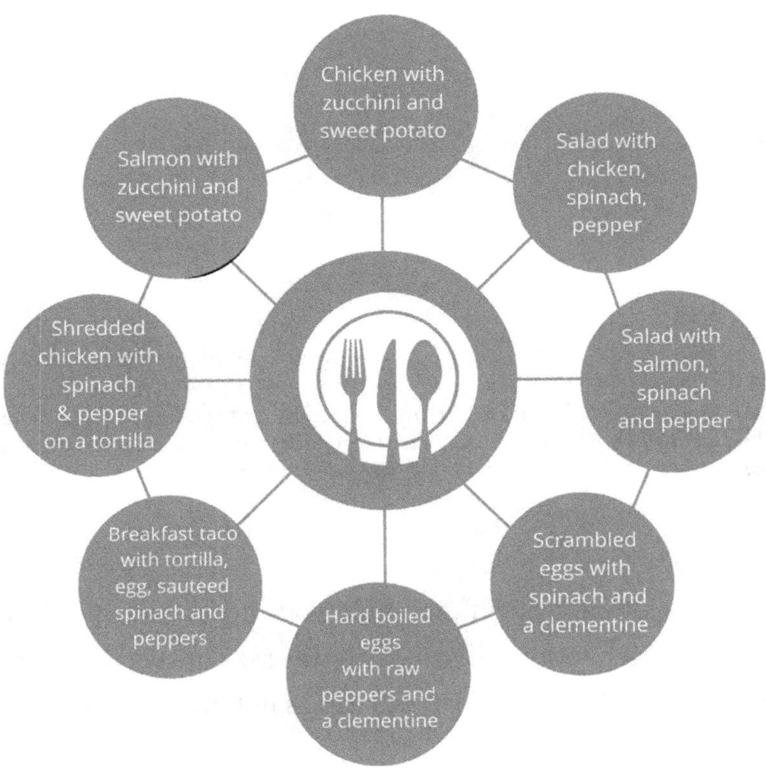

Diagram showing how the same or similar set of ingredients can be used to create a variety of meals.

After weight loss surgery, most bariatric patients can expect to lose anywhere from 60–77% of their excess body weight and maintain around 50% of that initial loss. This also equates to around 30–40% of total body weight loss.

I don't want anyone to mistake this for me saying that you "can't" hit a weight loss goal. Adjusting expectations doesn't mean you have to "settle" when it comes to your goals. I have full faith that you can do whatever you set your mind to. But the bigger question is, at what cost?

Your lowest weight is not always going to be your healthiest weight. Just like eating the smallest amount of food as possible for as long as possible isn't the goal, neither is trying to get as low as possible on the scale.

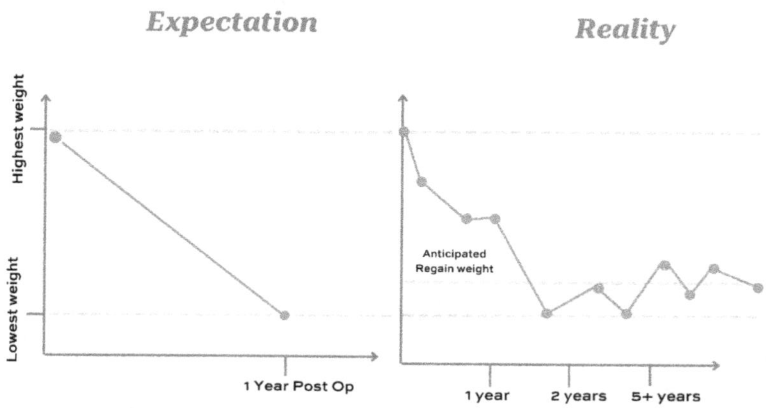

Line graph showing two different weight loss trends. The first is a hypothetical trajectory reflecting the expectation of rapid and consistent weight loss, and the second is the reality with weight loss slowly trending downwards over time and weight fluctuating.

If you have to "white-knuckle it" and fight your body, your mind, your cravings, and your hunger, tooth and nail, all for the sake of keeping the number as low as you can get it, I'm sorry, love, but that is not healthy or realistic.

Weight Fluctuations

First things first. Everyone's weight will fluctuate, whether you had surgery or not. So your scale went up 3 pounds overnight? Congratulations! You're a human!

So many people come to me in sheer and utter PANIC when this happens. Many of my DMs look a little something like this:

> *"OMG, Jamie, please help!! I have no idea what I'm doing wrong! I have*

been doing everything right, and I gained 3 lbs. since yesterday!!! How is that even possible?! Should I go back to liquids? Did I stretch my pouch? I feel like such a failure!"

When I get messages like this, I completely get and understand where this fear is coming from. But what I tell people who are struggling is this: *First, breathe! It's going to be okay. Second, your weight will shift from day to day.*

Some reasons for this include being dehydrated, being bloated, having more sodium the day before, having more carbs the day before (and no, for the hundredth time, carbs don't cause weight gain, they just cause our bodies to hold on to water), you haven't used the bathroom yet, you're stressed/inflamed, you have sore muscles, you're about to start your cycle, etc. Honestly? There's probably a hundred different reasons why your scale moved, and it's not always dependent on anything you did. So please, I beg you, stop unnecessarily beating yourself up!

<u>Stalls and Plateaus</u>

I'm going to throw some tough love at you right now (emphasis on the love, of course): just because you didn't lose weight today doesn't mean you are in a stall. If you haven't lost weight for a week, you are not in a stall. If you haven't lost weight for two weeks, you are not in a stall. Heck, if you haven't lost weight for three or four weeks, it doesn't necessarily mean you are in a stall.

The number on the scale is only one unit of measurement of progress. It doesn't show you the whole picture. Sometimes your body can still be changing, losing inches and losing fat mass, without the scale actually changing.

The thing is, if we are being realistic here, you will simply not lose weight every single week on this journey. That's not how weight loss works. Weight loss takes a lot of time and consistency. And even though you had weight loss surgery, which does usually result in quicker weight loss, it still doesn't mean the weight will magically fall off every time you get on the scale.

Not losing for days and weeks at a time is part of the weight loss process. And it's in those moments when you truly need to rely on being dedicated to your habits. Motivation is fleeting—meaning, you are not going to be motivated all of the time. And if you are solely using the number on the scale to motivate you, I'm sorry, love, but you are going to need to dig deeper than that. Because the scale simply will not always move.

And that doesn't mean you are doing anything wrong. When people don't lose weight for a bit, their knee-jerk reaction, again, is to beat themselves up, tell themselves they are failing, and convince themselves that they are broken or there must be something wrong with them.

One of the biggest mistakes I see when people are frustrated with the scale not moving is immediately "switching things up." Now, sometimes, if your body truly has adjusted to your routine, then you may need to "switch things up" or change something; but it's unlikely that's the case after just a few weeks of no weight loss. Rather than changing things, what people usually need is to be more consistent with what they already know they are supposed to be doing. When in doubt, focus on being CONSISTENT with your water and protein goal and see what happens. You usually don't need to change anything; you just need to keep doing the things you've already been doing. Sometimes what we need most is patience.

Weight Maintenance

One of the reasons I'm constantly telling people that they shouldn't use the scale alone for motivation is because, at some point on this journey, you WILL stop losing weight. You cannot keep losing weight forever. And sometimes, we are forced into maintenance sooner than maybe we would like.

But I want to remind you that maintenance in itself is such a HUGE win! For so many of us, we have always been on that "yo-yo" weight cycle of either losing or gaining. Being stable in your weight is a good thing. And sometimes, especially after extreme amounts of weight loss, we have to maintain for a bit in order to let our bodies adjust before we may be able to lose more weight again—if that's still something we are working towards. So if you've been maintaining your weight for a while now, even if that wasn't your goal, I want you to pause and give yourself a good pat on the back; because that's amazing.

Realistically, when it comes to maintenance, you are going to maintain within a range. Most people will maintain within 5–10 pounds or so. This is normal.

People always get anxious when it comes to weight maintenance, especially for those who have hit their goal weight. Many will ask, "What do I do now that I'm ready to maintain?"

And honestly? Your maintenance mode likely won't and shouldn't look too much different than when you were losing weight. Unless you are running the risk of losing too much, in which case you may need to strategically add more calories in (and if this is you, I suggest working with a dietitian on this), your maintenance routine won't look too different.

I tell people to focus less on maintaining their weight or the number on the scale and focus more on maintaining their habits. If you can continue with all the beautiful habits you've created during your weight loss stage, you likely will be able to maintain the majority of what you have lost. And since you will be able to eat more, if you are simply eating larger portions of the foods and food routines you've been sticking with all along, it's likely you will level out. This is another reason why building a realistic and sustainable routine that you actually enjoy is SO important. This is why I want people to fall in love with the process, not just the destination, from day one. Because if you enjoy the foods you eat and allow yourself flexibility and the opportunity to be consistent, it will be so much easier to maintain long term than if you are stuck in all-or-nothing thinking.

Rebound Weight vs. Regain

It's unrealistic to expect to stay at your lowest weight forever. But just because you have gone up on the scale doesn't mean you have "regained."

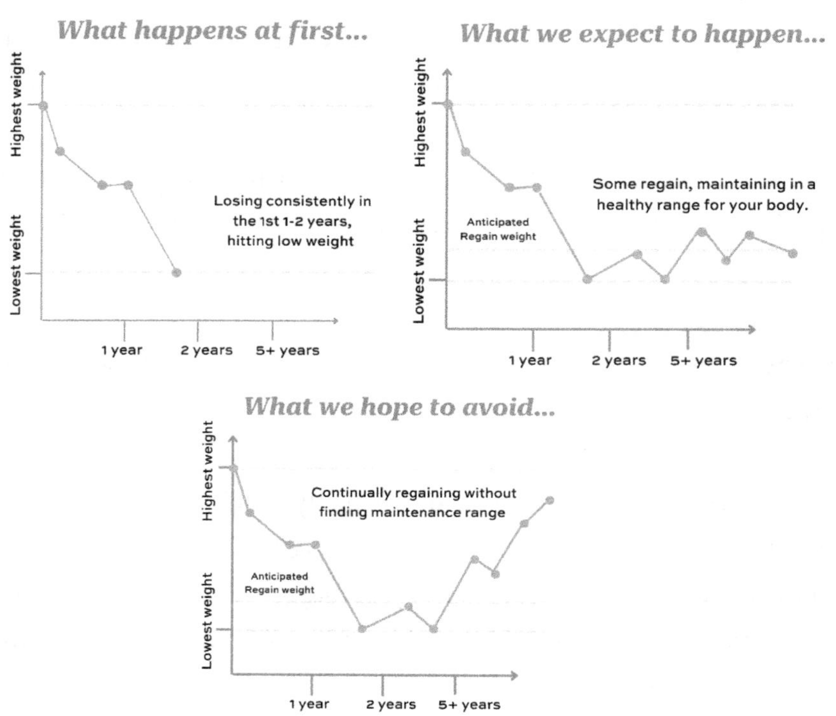

Line graph showing three different weight loss trends we expect to see over time as well as the regain trend we hope to avoid.

When I say "rebound" weight, I'm talking about that 10–17% or so of weight we expect to come back on over time. However, if you are dealing with weight gain beyond that, it's likely more of a true regain of weight rather than that anticipated rebound.

If you're struggling with regain, you are not alone. And there are ways to overcome it. (More on this to come in Chapter 11.)

Bite-Sized Recap

- Goals and routines after surgery need to be realistic.
- It's important to set realistic expectations in order to be consistent long term.
- Calorie and macro counting may be a great tool for some on their journeys, but for others it may promote all-or-nothing thinking.
- Nutrition-label reading is an important skill to have in order to better understand the foods you are consuming.
- It's not suggested to count net carbs after weight loss surgery.
- Meal planning does not have to be as hard or as tedious as some make it out to be. Work smarter not harder!
- Having realistic weight loss expectations is important.
- Stalls and plateaus will continue to happen throughout this journey and your weight will change and fluctuate.

For journal prompts related to this chapter and resources, such as my free bariatric meal planning guide, head to www.thesleeveddietitian.com/easy.

Chapter 9
The Bariatric Dos and Don'ts

rule

/ro͞ol/

noun

1. one of a set of explicit or understood regulations or principles governing conduct within a particular activity or sphere

"It's important to understand all the rules after surgery."

Our Inner Defiant Child

When I teach about the bariatric "rules" to my clients and in my programs, I like to refer to them as the "Bariatric Dos and Don'ts." I put the word "rules" in quotations, because I hate the idea that there are rules. The truth is, there are no rules. This is your life. This isn't a diet. This isn't a short-term fix. I think the idea of rules creates all-or-nothing thinking. While they aren't exactly "rules," they are guidelines set in place for safety and post-op success—each of which has their own set of potential consequences if not followed.

That being said, one of the biggest gaps in bariatric surgery education I see amongst bariatric patients is that they are so often told by their surgical team that they need to do these things after weight loss surgery, but are never told WHY. If you're never told what those consequences could be, how are you supposed to make an educated and informed decision for yourself to follow what you've been told?

I don't know about you, but when I'm told "you need to do this" or "you can't do that," my immediate subconscious response is defiance. If someone says "don't touch the red button," what do you want to do? You want to touch the red button. We can't help it. No one likes being told what to do. And for bariatric patients, most have been on fad diets their whole lives, dictated by these arbitrary rules set up by diet culture that actually make no sense—"Don't eat carbs" or "Don't eat after 7:00 p.m." There's no science behind either of those rules. They make no sense.

But because there is such a lack of proper nutrition education in our society as a whole, in a world where 15-year-old Tik Tok influencers are selling green juice or where "fitness gurus" with 100K followers on Instagram can sell you their garbage meal plans with no repercussions, how is anyone without a science or nutrition background supposed to decipher between the pseudoscience and the real recommendations?

After surgery, if you don't stick to the bariatric rules and guidelines, the implications go beyond simply just not hitting your weight loss goal. Failing to follow the bariatric rules can lead to serious repercussions, complications, and consequences because of the way your anatomy has been changed.

There's also this common fear amongst bariatric patients that they are going to "stretch their pouch" out—their pouch meaning their "new" stomach. This fear runs very deep. It's not just a fear of "ruining" their new stomach, but the fear that they somehow will "fail."

I personally can relate to this. Years of chronic dieting absolutely contribute to all-or-nothing thinking. This thinking often carries over post-op. It's the fear that you make one "wrong" move or decision, that you somehow "ruined" everything and have "failed." That on-again-off-again mentality. As a perfectionist and people pleaser, I too have had to work really hard to get out of that type of thinking. And it doesn't happen overnight.

While there are things we need to do after bariatric surgery, and some rules can cause immediate consequences, how do we teach these patients the "rules" while also getting them out of this black-and-white thinking? Well, it starts with education. It starts with doing the following:

1. Explaining what they should be doing;
2. Explaining what they should not be doing;
3. Explaining the consequences that could occur if they don't follow through;
4. Supporting, educating, and encouraging them to want to make these changes for themselves, not for anyone else or simply because you said so.

And to all my bariatricians and colleagues whose reasoning is "because I said so"— as practitioners, we can and NEED to do better than that. Instead, let's help our patients understand the reasons behind what we are asking them to do. Below is the list of standard bariatric "rules" that most surgical centers implement and how I explain these changes to my own clients, so they can feel empowered to implement these changes with confidence. In my explanations, I also dispel myths surrounding these recommendations.

The Don'ts: The Things You Should Avoid, Limit, or Eliminate After Weight Loss Surgery to Avoid Complications and to Achieve Long-Term Success

Below are some of the most common rules that bariatric patients are advised to not do. In this section, I share with you what the rule is and why some surgeons advise it.

Don't Drink Through a Straw

There are two main reasons why you should avoid drinking through straws immediately after surgery. The first is because straws can lead to "chugging" your water or fluids. The reason you don't want to chug is it can make you feel very sick and uncomfortable after surgery. Your new stomach is very small, and drinking too quickly will fill your stomach too fast, leading to potential nausea and vomiting. The second reason is because the use of the straw can cause air bubbles to get caught in your belly, which can cause pain, discomfort, and/or belching.

All that being said, one of the biggest misconceptions is that drinking through a straw will cause you to "stretch your pouch" (i.e., your stomach). This is false. The air bubbles will not cause harm beyond some discomfort and will not stretch out your surgically created or altered stomach. And with that in mind, some bariatric patients argue that using a straw actually helps them to meet their hydration goals. So what I tell my clients is if straws don't cause discomfort, and they don't enable you to chug your fluids, from a clinical standpoint, there really is no reason for you to have to stick to this particular "don't" long term. Knowing the potential benefits and consequences of the straw usage, it's up to you what you choose to do.

Don't Drink Carbonated Beverages

I'll be honest, I was pretty devastated when I learned that I had to give up my beloved seltzer water after surgery. This is another "bariatric rule" a lot of people aren't aware of. Carbonated beverages include seltzer waters, soda (both diet and regular), fizzy alcohol, and kombucha. Aside from the calories and sugar content in sodas and alcohol (see more details on this below), carbonation has a similar effect on bariatric patients to that of straws. The carbonation can cause air bubbles that cause pain and discomfort.

But just like with straws, it is a myth (at least to my knowledge) that the carbonation can stretch your stomach. Many patients are led to believe that this is a consequence of drinking carbonation. However, I have yet to see a research study that determines this is the case. So please, if you know of a reliable research study that suggests otherwise, send it my way. But until then, I don't believe there is evidence to support the claim that carbonation can do damage to your pouch.

However, all that being said, SO many bariatric patients struggle with soda addictions pre-surgery. If drinking carbonation from seltzer water or diet soda, although calorie- and sugar-free, might trigger you or be a gateway to going back to full-sugar soda, I strongly caution you against choosing to add that back into your routine. But if soda isn't a trigger for you, I don't think there's a reason to avoid it life long unless you personally choose to.

No Eating and Drinking Together

This is easily one of the hardest bariatric habits to get used to. Most surgical centers suggest spacing out eating and drinking together by 30 minutes. So that usually means after you take a sip of water/fluid, you have to wait 30 minutes from that last sip until you can eat your food.

Most suggest taking 20–30 minutes to eat your meal slowly (see below for more details). Once you are done with that last bite of food, you then are told to wait another 30 minutes before you can resume sipping your fluids. A sample eating and drinking schedule might look like this:

- 9:00–9:30 a.m.: slowly sip water
- 9:30–10:00 a.m.: stop eating and drinking
- 10:00–10:30 a.m.: slowly eat your breakfast
- 10:30–11:00 a.m.: stop eating and drinking
- 11:00–11:30 a.m.: resume sipping water

This concept might sound wild and very strange if it's the first time you're hearing it. The reason bariatric patients are told to do this is because if you drink too closely to eating, you can fill up your pouch with fluid, making it more difficult to eat your meal and get your nutrition needs met. On the flip side, after you eat, you don't want to drink too soon; because your stomach is already full, and there usually isn't room to fit those fluids into your pouch as the food is digesting. Drinking too soon after eating can cause pain and discomfort, dumping syndrome (more on this in the next few pages), and possible vomiting.

One of the rebuttals I hear often to this bariatric "don't" is this: "Well, Jamie, eating and drinking together doesn't bother me. I can tolerate it just fine." Ah, okay, valid point there. Some bariatric patients CAN fit both fluids and solid food into their pouch at the same time. But just because you can, doesn't mean you should.

When you eat and drink together after weight loss surgery, the fluid pushes the food you've just eaten through your pouch more quickly. Picture a funnel. Imagine that you put applesauce in that funnel. It will very slowly drip out of the bottom. Now envision pouring water on top of that applesauce that was slowly dripping out. What will happen if you pour water on top of that applesauce is the water will force it through the funnel more quickly. The same exact thing happens when you drink and eat together after bariatric surgery. Because of this, if you flush out the food that is in your stomach, you are going to create more space for more food. This is one of the "bariatric loopholes," as I like to call it. It's a way to eat around that tight restriction one feels when they have surgery. In turn, you are able to create more space to eat more, thus defeating the purpose of your smaller stomach. One of the habits I often see amongst bariatric patients experiencing significant regain is the habit of eating and drinking together as a regular part of their routine.

Don't Drink Sugar-Sweetened Beverages

Sugar-sweetened beverages (sodas, juices, sweetened teas and coffees, energy drinks, etc.) are one of the leading causes of type 2 diabetes and contributors to heart disease, both comorbidities of obesity. Sugar-sweetened beverages can add a significant amount of calories and sugar to your day, which can certainly contribute to weight gain and obesity. I want to give you some real-life context for how this can actually manifest in your day-to-day life.

Let's talk about a 16-ounce can bottle of Coke, for example. One 16-ounce bottle is approximately 200 calories and 52 grams of sugar. Every 4 grams of sugar is the equivalent of 1 teaspoon. So in this one bottle of Coke, you are taking in approximately 13 teaspoons of sugar—the recommended daily allowance. The American Heart Association recommends no more than 9 teaspoons of sugar per day for men and no more than 6 teaspoons per day for women.[94]

Let's make that even a bit more relatable. Sugar content aside, drinking 16 ounces of Coke adds about 200 calories to your day—not that much, to be completely honest. And for the record, calories are NOT the enemy. Calories are a unit of energy that our body needs in order to survive, and lower calorie is not always better. However, where our calories come from matters, and 200 calories of liquid is not going to fill you up or keep you full.

That 200 calories can add up quickly. Let's do some math, shall we? Let's say you have just one 16-ounce bottle of Coke per day each day.

200 calories x 365 days per year = 73,000 calories per year

Okay, cool, but how does that correlate to weight?

Every one pound of fat is approximately 3,500 calories. So if we take 73,000 calories per year from Coke alone and divide it by 3,500, that equals 20.8 pounds. So theoretically, if all you did was cut out that one soda per day, technically you should lose nearly 21 pounds in a year. I say theoretically because, as always, there are lots of nuances that feed into this equation and LOTS of factors that play into the "calories in versus calories out" equation. But you get the picture. Calories from sugar that lead to other diseases and don't fill us up are just simply not ideal, and if you are someone who struggles with sugar or soda addiction, it can be a very slippery slope.

In addition, sugar-sweetened beverages can also lead to something called "dumping syndrome." **Dumping syndrome** is a condition in which foods that are high in sugar, and sometimes fat, move through your stomach to your

[94] "Get the Facts: Added Sugars," "Nutrition: Diet & Statistics" section of CDC website, last updated November 28, 2021, https://www.cdc.gov/nutrition/data-statistics/added-sugars.html.

small intestines too quickly after you eat or drink, which often happens as a result of surgery on your stomach.[95]

Dumping syndrome probably isn't what you think (no, it's not having uncontrollable bowel movements). Rather, it's a full-body effect that can happen anywhere from 10 minutes to up to three hours after you've consumed something high in sugar and/or fat. The influx of sugar concentration that enters into your small intestine can result in nausea, vomiting, abdominal cramping, rapid heart rate, labored breathing, weakness, vomiting, and in some cases, diarrhea. Usually people experience either all of these things at once or a combination of these things.

Patients are often told that only those who have RNY or DS can experience dumping syndrome. Ah, but alas, as someone with VSG, I can assure you that is, in fact, false. While not everyone with VSG will experience dumping syndrome, I am one of the "lucky ones," as I like to joke, who has experienced this multiple times since my surgery. For me, it feels like a sudden panic attack combined with the intense urge to vomit and use the bathroom. It is quite unpleasant.

Again, all of these bariatric rules are not simply for weight loss results, but for your safety and health as a result of your anatomy changing. Do with these recommendations what you will, but don't say I didn't tell you so! I like to think dumping syndrome is a "live and learn experience." (Fun sidenote: ice cream is REALLY good at causing dumping syndrome. Proceed with caution.)

Don't Consume Alcohol

Every bariatric center has a slightly different stance on alcohol, although most will suggest removing alcohol from your life for at least a year post-op. This is

---

[95] "Dumping Syndrome," "Diseases & Conditions" section of Mayo Clinic website, last updated June 17, 2022, https://www.mayoclinic.org/diseases-conditions/dumping-syndrome/symptoms-causes/syc-20371915.

what I recommend to my own clients. There are a multitude of reasons why alcohol should be avoided after weight loss surgery.

For starters, like soda, many alcoholic beverages add additional sugars and calories to your routine in liquid form that will not keep you full.

Alcohol is also dehydrating. As bariatric patients, it can be especially difficult to stay hydrated after surgery. As you just learned, you aren't supposed to eat and drink together, so working toward your hydration needs can be very difficult and time-consuming. The last thing you want to do is further put yourself at risk for dehydration.

Alcohol is also intoxicating. Did you know that post-op, you can become intoxicated much more quickly? Because your stomach capacity is so much smaller, the surface area of your stomach is smaller, allowing for much quicker and faster absorption of alcohol into the bloodstream, resulting in one becoming much more intoxicated off lesser amounts of alcohol than they might be used to. For example, half a glass of wine will for sure make me tipsy. My husband jokes I'm a cheap date. (Full disclosure: at this point in my journey, I do enjoy alcohol moderately in my routine, but it was not something I was able to do in the beginning of my journey.)

Because you can get intoxicated much more quickly after weight loss surgery, you have the potential to be a risk to yourself and others. Think about it. If you're out with friends and don't realize that just a few sips of wine will make you drunk, you may unintentionally get behind the wheel without realizing just how intoxicated you are. You never want to put yourself or others in dangerous situations.

And lastly, alcohol consumption can lead to what's called a "transfer addiction" after weight loss surgery. Not all, but many, bariatric patients struggle with some form of emotional eating, binge eating, coping with food, and/or food addiction. While there is some controversy surrounding the topic of "food addictions" (some say it's impossible to be addicted to something you need to live), I do think it's fair to say that many who struggle with their weight and their relationship with food have addictive personality types or traits, as well as difficulty coping with trauma and emotions. When a normal coping mechanism (food, in this example) is removed, people often turn to other addictions to fill that void. Some of these addictions might look like shopping or gambling. But for others, it could very easily become alcohol. The repercussions of this could be devastating, if not fatal.

You should always follow your surgery center's guidelines and recommendations when it comes to introducing alcohol back into your routine, and I strongly suggest doing so, if and when you are ready, alongside the care of a credentialed and licensed mental health professional.

Don't Consume Caffeine

Much like alcohol, caffeine can be dehydrating. It's a natural diuretic, which means it promotes the excretion of the fluids and water in your body. In our bodies, we have a hormone called antidiuretic hormone (also known as ADH) that helps regulate the water in our bodies and filters the fluids through our kidneys to be excreted as urine. Caffeine triggers ADH. And while fluid losses from caffeine may be minimal and not majorly impactful on the average person, it's already challenging enough to stay hydrated at baseline after surgery. Not to mention, dehydration combined with a mostly protein diet (see below) has the potential to put strain on your kidneys, which is another reason staying hydrated is so important. I would always rather bariatric patients err on the side of caution when it comes to caffeine so they aren't putting themselves at higher risk for potential dehydration.

Now friends, please do not panic. I myself am a self-proclaimed coffee connoisseur. To say I love coffee would be an understatement. Before you shudder at my next suggestion, I want to remind you that this journey is a lot of give and take. There are things, unfortunately, that we must sacrifice. So while it pains my coffee-loving heart to type these words, I would suggest switching to a decaf coffee option, until at least the first 9–12 months post-op. Decaf coffee can give you that coffee-lover's fix while also helping you hit your fluid goals. One of the things I tell my clients is that once you are consistently hitting your protein goal, then it should be okay to add a bit of caffeine back in. But as always, please check with your surgeon or personal dietitian before doing so. Caffeine also has the potential to cause stomach ulcers and gastrointestinal (GI) discomfort, so it's important to introduce caffeine back into your diet with the guidance of your own team.

Don't Eat Past Your Fullness Cues

This is a big one. And a hard one. While you have surgery on your stomach, unfortunately, you do not have surgery on your brain. While most bariatric patients can pretty intensely feel the sensation of fullness after weight loss surgery (I interchangeably refer to fullness after bariatric surgery as "your restriction"), it does not always leave one feeling satisfied. It can be incredibly frustrating to take two or three bites of food and feel full. It often takes the enjoyment out of food. But friends, that is partly the point. It's not that you can never enjoy food again, but it's so important to utilize your tool as it was intended in order to make sure you stop when you're feeling full.

One of the ways I suggest increasing your satisfaction is to make sure you are taking your time with your meals, eating slowly, and really practicing being mindful. That usually means savoring each bite and not eating while distracted.

One of the biggest fears amongst the bariatric community is of "stretching your pouch out." So many bariatric patients that I speak to tell me that when they eat that one bite too many or push their restriction, they immediately worry that they will "stretch" their pouch or "ruin everything."

I'm excited to share that's next to impossible. One extra bite here and there is not going to cause your stomach to stretch. It's just not possible. But what it will do is cause discomfort, maybe nausea, and possible vomiting.

Over time, you WILL be able to eat more volume of food. This is normal. The stomach is a muscle, and as time goes on after surgery and your internal incisions heal and swelling subsides, your stomach does stretch a bit and regains that elasticity that muscles naturally have.

Knowing that you will be able to eat more again over time, it's even more important to make sure you are stopping as soon as you feel full. Otherwise, that one bite too many can turn to many more bites. In later chapters, I talk more about the nuances and reasons why some people push their restriction, eat past their fullness, and struggle to stick to this rule. It's much easier said than done, and if you struggle with this, you are not alone. But it is still something I really encourage you to practice.

Don't Skip Post-Op Diet Stages

Time for some tough love (emphasis on the love). Your post-op diet prescribed to you by your bariatric team is there for a reason. It's not up for interpretation, and it is not optional. It is 100% there for your safety and success on this journey. Is it hard to follow a diet? Yes. Yes it is. This is one of the reasons why preoperative nutrition counseling is so important; there should be no surprises of what's expected of you after surgery.

For the first 4–6 weeks post-op, most bariatric patients have some type of slow diet progression in terms of the texture of their diet. Usually, this looks like slowly advancing through clear liquids, full liquids, pureed foods, soft foods, and then solid foods.

This is here for your safety. I cannot stress this enough. Right after surgery, you have internal incisions that are healing. Skipping stages can be incredibly dangerous. You run the risk of tearing your internal wounds and causing a leak or perforation.

The Dos: The Things You Should Implement, Practice, and Build Your Routines Around, for a Successful and Sustainable Weight Loss Surgery Journey

Below are some of the most common practices that bariatric patients are advised to follow. In this section, I share with you what the rule is and why it's important.

Do Follow Your Prescribed Post-Op Diet

Not only are bariatric patients given a post-op diet in terms of texture, but most are given very specific instruction on what foods they should and shouldn't be eating, even after they hit the solid-food stage.

This is where it gets tricky. Every surgical center seems to provide slightly different post-op diets. In general, though, these diets are usually high in protein and fiber and lower in refined carbs and fat. I want to stress this here, again, very clearly: carbohydrates and fats are not bad. There are no such things as "good" or "bad" foods. However, foods do provide different nutrient compositions and are processed differently in the body.

Do Hit Your Protein Goals

When one undergoes extreme weight loss, it's inevitable that they are going to lose both fat and muscle tissue. The goal is to preserve as much as much of that muscle tissue as possible, and one does this by eating adequate protein.

When you don't get adequate protein, your body still needs the amino acids from those proteins in order for your body to function properly. So if you don't consume enough protein, you will break down your own muscle and draw from your body's stores. Not only does not eating enough protein lead to potential malnutrition, but it also is not desirable for maintaining long-term weight loss results. When this happens, your BMR (basal metabolic rate, i.e., the calories you burn at rest) lowers, making it even harder to sustain your weight loss as time goes on.

It's not that bariatric patients need to eat more protein than the average person; it's just that their portion sizes are so small that protein needs to take priority when being consumed. I usually suggest to my clients to make at least half of their plate protein, or aim for at least 3 ounces of lean protein per meal.

This is the reason bariatric patients end up with such a high-protein, low-carb diet after weight loss surgery. It's not that the other foods are "bad," it's that protein has to take priority. And while everyone's portions are different, and your portions will increase over time, it's not unusual to be eating 3–5 ounces total per meal in the beginning. And if you're focusing on 3 ounces of protein to hit your goal, well, that doesn't leave a ton of room for much else.

Do Hit Your Fiber Goals

Fiber, as we already learned, helps keep you fuller longer and slows down digestion. Not only is fiber important for keeping you fuller longer, but it's also incredibly important for overall heart health, cholesterol, and digestion. Many bariatric patients also suffer from constipation after surgery. Increasing both fiber and water can really benefit you with this struggle. If you struggle with hitting your fiber goal from foods alone, talk to your surgeon or dietitian about potentially adding in a fiber supplement if needed and if allowed.

Do Hit Your Fluid Goals and Sip Slowly

We've already talked a lot about the potential risks for dehydration and why it's so important to be mindful of fluids. The general recommendation is 64 ounces of fluid per day. I tell my clients that any noncarbonated, sugar-free, nonalcoholic, noncaffeinated beverage counts toward their water intake. Personally, I really struggle with just plain water since surgery. In order for me to hit my water goal, even all these years out, I rely pretty heavily on flavored options like sugar-free Gatorade and Crystal Light.

Do Take Your Vitamins

Just like not getting enough protein can lead to malnutrition, the same goes for not taking adequate vitamins after bariatric surgery. Since your food intakes are so limited after surgery, it's very challenging to get all of the micronutrients your body needs from foods alone. Not to mention, if you have a malabsorptive surgery (such as RNY, DS, or SADI-S), you will not absorb all the micronutrients you consume.

Even after having VSG, which is not considered malabsorptive, it's important to take bariatric-formulated vitamins long term. Some nutrients, such as B12, are absorbed in the stomach. It's important that you are still getting adequate supplementation.

One of the common misconceptions I hear from people is that they can stop taking their vitamins as long as their bloodwork comes back normal. This is false, my friend. It's likely the reason your bloodwork is normal is because you are taking your supplements. Nutrient deficiencies, some of which can be detrimental to your health, likely won't show up on your bloodwork until years 3–5 post-op. You don't want to run the risk of needing iron infusions or B12 shots after surgery. Nutrient deficiencies also can lead to bone density loss, teeth loss, and hair loss. I get it; I know taking vitamins sucks. But it's a necessary evil.

The Importance of Understanding the WHY Behind the Rules

After weight loss surgery, you need to understand which habits you need to adapt to fully and why. Weight loss surgery patients need to be able to take these habits and implement them long term into their new lives. And I know these rules might seem overwhelming at first. They are. It's a whole new world to get used to. But you can do hard things. And with a little education, encouragement, and a sprinkle of creativity, it is totally possible to ENJOY your routine by making the things you love more bariatric friendly.

Nothing aggravates me more than when someone comes to me and says, "My surgery center told me to do this, but I don't know why." As both a practitioner and a patient myself, this is infuriating. As clinicians, how do we expect people to stick to what we're telling them if they are going into this blindly and have no idea why they're being instructed to do the things you say? As a patient, how are you supposed to remember each and every one of these dos and don'ts if none of it makes any sense?

One of the other things I hear from people is, "I know my surgery center told me to do x, y, and z; but I just can't for x, y, and z reasons. I feel like a failure." If your patient expresses to you that they are struggling with committing to a habit change, it's your job as the practitioner to work with them on the barriers they are facing. It's your job to figure out a way to support them in making habits that are doable and achievable. And if they aren't able to stick to the habits that are set in place for their ultimate safety, then you shouldn't be approving them for surgery to begin with, at least not until they are fully confident they can stick to the program guideline afterwards.

When I was in the pre-op stage myself, I remember one specific conversation I had with my own dietitian. Let me preface this by saying that I adored her, and she was absolutely wonderful. But I did disagree with her.

I was sitting across from her at her desk, reviewing my post-op diet instructions with her. As we moved through the liquid, puree, soft food, and solid food stages together, and what was allowed at each stage, I asked her some specific questions about protein bars.

"I noticed that protein bars aren't allowed on my post-op-diet at all, even once I'm back to solid foods. Since I'll be at my internship rotations for very long hours, would it be okay if sometimes, in a pinch, I had a protein bar? I know some of them are really high in protein and low-carb, so they have similar nutrition in them to a protein shake."

"Well . . . protein shakes are fine. But not protein bars," she replied hesitantly.

"How come?" I asked.

"Well . . . so it's not that the protein bars are bad. They're fine actually. But the reason we don't allow them on the post-op diet at all is because most bariatric patients don't understand the difference between protein bars and candy bars. And we don't want them eating candy bars."

I sat there and blinked at her, dumbfounded.

She continued, "But you're not like all our other patients, and I know you understand nutrition since you're in school to be a dietitian. So I don't mind making the exception. Since you know the difference, I think it would be fine if you had one once in a while."

Ummm . . . I'm sorry . . . WHAT?! There was so much to unpack and pick apart here. Which, don't worry, I will continue to do throughout the entirety of this book. Here's the thing: if your bariatric patient truly doesn't know the difference between a Snickers bar and protein bar, it's YOUR job as the dietitian to educate them. To sit down and explain the nutrient differences. To teach them how to label read. And if they aren't grasping those concepts, then it's probably not the best idea to push them along in the surgical process; because, clearly, they need more time for education sessions.

What really bothers me with this, more than anything, is the stereotyping. Why are we assuming that weight loss surgery patients can't distinguish a protein bar from a candy bar? Because once again, we are faced with the unfortunate stigmas attached to bariatric surgery patients: That they don't care to try hard enough. That they are going to be noncompliant with what you tell them regardless. That "fat" people are lazy and stupid. It's this idea that, even if you told them the "why" behind a "rule," they aren't going to follow it anyway; so rather than allowing them to make an empowered decision for themselves, you just tell them "no," because you don't trust that they are smart or able enough to make the healthful choice to begin with.

THIS is why it's so important to me to not just tell you what the bariatric rules are, but WHY they should be followed.

Again, I truly did love the dietitian I worked with at my weight loss surgery center. She was caring and kind, and I felt like she was genuinely rooting for me. And her whole job is to help bariatric patients lose weight and get healthier. And even still, she too wasn't above the stigmas our society has surrounding individuals in bigger bodies, whether she was even aware of it or not.

Her not wanting her patients to have protein bars out of fear they would mistake them for candy bars is a classic example of assuming that, just because one lives in a larger body, they must not be *competent* enough to critically think through that decision-making process.

You can't expect someone to change or make a new habit if they have no idea why they are doing it in the first place. So why aren't all bariatric centers teaching their patients the how tos and the whys of these rules?

So if you are a practitioner and you are reading this, I want to empower you to teach your patients the *why* behind your recommendation. Teach them what they need to know to be successful, and set the expectation that you believe in them to make the changes they need to, and guide them as they rise to the occasion. Because I promise you, if you simply tell them "no" without explanation, you will be doing them a huge disservice.

And if you are reading this as a bariatric patient I want to encourage and empower you to ask questions during your office visits. If you are told you can't have something after surgery or that you shouldn't do something, I want you to advocate for yourself and ask why that is. Not to argue with your team, but so that you can take ownership in your journey and truly understand what changes YOU need to make and why.

Bite-Sized Recap

- Having bariatric surgery comes with its own set of unique rules.
- It's important to understand the why behind these rules so that you can make empowered decisions surrounding how you follow and implement these rules into your own routine.
- As bariatric patients, some of the "don'ts" include eating and drinking together, using straws, drinking carbonated beverages, consuming sugar-sweetened beverages, alcohol, and caffeine.
- As bariatric patients, some of the "dos" include following your post-op diet; hitting your protein, fiber, and fluid goals; and taking your vitamins.

For journal prompts and resources related to this chapter be sure to head to www.thesleeveddietitian.com/easy.

Chapter 10
What I Wish I Knew: My Top Tips for Navigating Life After Surgery

ad·vice

/əd'vaɪs/

noun

1. guidance or recommendations offered with regard to prudent future action

"She wanted all the advice she could get to reach her goals."

There's no right or wrong way to navigate post-surgery life.

When I was awaiting my VSG surgery date, I was like a sponge, ready to absorb every bit of advice and information I could get. I was going to do this "right," and I was determined to be successful.

Since I didn't know anyone in my life at the time who had had surgery, the only place I thought to go to for advice was Facebook. At the time, I thought it was helpful, since I was able to hear other people's experiences and suggestions. But what I soon realized was that there were a lot of people giving advice that was either unsolicited or blatantly incorrect. It caused a lot of confusion, and oftentimes, it seemed to spark more anxiety for me than it helped. The advice given to those who asked questions in the forums felt a lot more like critiques and passing judgment than actual help.

They say you should never take criticism from someone you wouldn't take advice from, and I think that's important to remember. It's also important to remember that there is no one right or wrong way to navigate post-surgery life and to hit your goals.

If you feel like you need advice on your journey, I'd like to share with you the answers to all the questions I once had, in case you too, feel like you have nowhere to go to ask your questions and hear from someone who "gets it." If you feel alone on your journey, if you feel scared and overwhelmed, and if you feel like you need a good pep talk or some encouragement, say no more! Consider me your Bariatric Big Sister. I got you.

But also keep in mind that the advice I give you here is based on my own experiences as both a professional and patient, but that still doesn't mean everything I suggest is going to work for you. I encourage you to take these tidbits of advice and apply what feels right for you to your own routine.

In this chapter, I'm going to answer the most common questions I get asked, as well as the questions I once had. My answers to these questions are a combination of evidence-based answers and my personal opinion based on my lived experiences. It's everything I wish I knew and had answers to when I was first getting ready to embark on this journey.

"What should I pack for my hospital stay? How should I prepare for surgery?"

It's normal to feel anxious before your surgery and getting ready for your hospital stay. I often see people make the mistake of packing too much for their stay; remember, you will be very sleepy and spend your time recovering. You also will most likely only be there one or two nights.

I suggest packing very comfy/loose fitting pajamas or comfy clothes, an extra long phone charger, a comfy pillow from home (only if you prefer it), and ChapStick (your mouth will likely be dry when you wake up, and you may not be able to try sipping water for a little bit).

But honestly? That's really it! You're probably not going to have time to read that book you brought or need all those toiletries. The hospital typically gives you a toothbrush and toothpaste, as well as grippy socks for walking up and down the halls (so you probably don't need slippers either).

If it's allowed, I might suggest packing your own preferred protein shake and perhaps a sugar-free Gatorade and/or some Crystal Light or water enhancer. This may not be allowed, but if it is, it can be helpful for when they have you try clear and/or full liquids in the hospital. Oftentimes the hospitals only carry Ensure or Boost protein shakes (neither of which I preferred), and sometimes they don't have anything but plain water for clear liquids.

In addition, I would recommend cleaning your house and putting fresh sheets on your bed before you leave for your surgery. You are going to be tired when you get home, and it's much nicer to relax in a clean home than feeling like you have a million things to do. I also suggest taking anything you might need during recovery down from high shelves, as reaching up to grab things can put pressure on your incisions.

"Any suggestions for the liquid and puree food stage?"

My number one suggestion is to not stock up on too many protein shakes before surgery. Your tastes will change, and oftentimes, the protein shakes you enjoyed before you may not enjoy after.

Follow your surgery centers guidelines EXACTLY as they are laid out for you on paper, and if you have any questions, be sure to call and ask your dietitian or surgeon. The post-op diet isn't a suggestion, and it's not up for interpretation. If you are not able to eat soft or solid foods yet, DO NOT advance to other food textures before you are cleared to do so. This isn't for weight loss; this is for your safety. If you progress before you are medically cleared, you run the risk of severe complications. You have to remember that you have internal stitches that need time to heal.

Your options on the liquid and puree stages will be boring. I get asked a lot, "Do you have any good recipes or ways to switch it up?" on liquids and puree. And my honest answer? No, unfortunately I don't. Liquids and purees *are* boring. You're very limited on what you can have. Most surgery centers allow protein shakes, yogurt, cottage cheese, ricotta bake, low-fat refried beans, and pureed chicken/tuna salad. It's not super exciting. But some honest truth? It's not supposed to be. In addition to having a limited/bland diet so you can heal, you also should be capitalizing on this time to emotionally distance and remove yourself from food. So I will tell you what no one else will: it's okay if it's not fun. As time goes on, you will be able to add more back in, just not right away.

"I'm 3 weeks post-op, and I haven't lost any weight. Is this normal?"

Ah yes, the infamous three-week stall. Stalls will happen this entire time, and many people experience a stall between weeks 3–5 post-op. Your body is healing, and it's completely normal. For more on navigating stalls, head to Chapter 8.

"I feel like a failure because I'm not losing as quickly as others or as quickly as I thought I would. How am I ever going to hit my goal?"

One step at a time, my friend, one step at a time! You did not gain all of the weight in one day, and you will not lose it all at once either. Everyone's body is different, and each person will lose at their own pace. I know it's easier said than done, but try not to compare your journey to others'. You could have the same surgery date, starting weight, and surgery type as someone, and the two of you would still lose differently. My best advice is to keep going. Giving up on yourself just because it is slower than you imagined isn't going to get you to your goals any quicker. You're allowed to be annoyed or even disappointed that it's taking longer than you thought, but trust the process, follow your plan, and be consistent. The weight loss will follow.

"Is the bariatric diet the same for all bariatric patients?"

Yes and no. The overall bariatric guidelines are the same between all the surgery types, and my bariatric meal plate method and nutrition info I teach here in this book and to my clients is appropriate for all bariatric surgery types. Some surgeries do have some things they need to be aware of, especially when it comes to sugar and fat content if you have a malabsorptive surgery.

The confusing thing is though, every bariatric center will have slightly different post-op diet philosophies, so it's important to follow YOUR post-op diet versus comparing it to someone else's. If you have questions about your post-op diet, be sure to reach out to your surgery center and schedule an appointment with your dietitian.

"What's dumping syndrome?"

Dumping syndrome is a condition where foods, especially food high in sugar, moves from your stomach into your small bowel too quickly after you eat. It's also called "rapid gastric emptying."[96] This can happen as a result of bariatric surgery. While dumping syndrome occurs most often in RNY patients, it is a myth that VSG and other bariatric patients can't have dumping syndrome, even if it's less likely. One of the reasons I chose to have VSG over RNY was because I didn't want to experience this, but to my great surprise, I'm one of the few VSG patients who gets dumping syndrome if I'm not careful with my food choices.

Dumping syndrome usually occurs 10–30 minutes after eating something high in sugar and/or fat. This can especially happen if you have a liquid that is high in sugar and fat, such as a milkshake or ice cream, or if you eat and drink together.

Despite its name, dumping syndrome isn't just needing to use the bathroom. Signs and symptoms of dumping syndrome usually include full-body symptoms like rapid heart rate, flushing, sweating, dizziness/weakness, nausea, ab-

[96] Mayo Clinic, "Dumping Syndrome."

dominal cramps, diarrhea, and/or vomiting.

For me, when I experience dumping syndrome, I get incredibly overwhelmed and panicky, a racing heartbeat, sweating, and I get intensely nauseous as well as having abdominal cramping. I will say, it is unpleasant enough that I no longer attempt to eat the foods that I know cause it for me, as it's just not worth it.

"How often should I be exercising?/ What are the best exercises to do after surgery?"

The best exercise is the one you will stick to consistently. There is no right or wrong exercise. Find something you enjoy! And bonus points if you find something that is a combination of weight training and cardio. The standard recommendation is 30 minutes per day, but personally, I don't think that's realistic for everyone. I would recommend starting "small," even if that's just 10 minutes of walking per day, and to keep increasing and building from there.

"Can I still be a vegetarian/vegan after WLS?"

Totally! But unless you are a vegan/vegetarian before surgery, I wouldn't suggest becoming one after surgery. There's a lot of misconceptions about plant-based diets. I think they are particularly challenging for bariatric patients because it can be very challenging to meet your protein needs if you are not consuming meat, poultry, fish, eggs, and/or dairy products. It's also incredibly important to make sure you are getting the proper vitamin supplementation if you are vegetarian or vegan (to be clear it's important for ALL bariatric patients, but if you are following a plant-based diet, you are at even higher risk for nutrient deficiencies).

"What can I do to avoid loose skin and hair loss after surgery?"

The reality is, most people are going to experience some hair loss and loose skin after weight loss surgery. Unless you have incredible genes, loose skin is really hard to avoid. But there are some things you can do to help reduce the amount of loose skin you have and the hair you may lose.

Loose skin suggestions: Try to make sure you are incorporating strength training into your routine early on in your journey. If you can maintain muscle mass on your body, it can help with the loose skin. Keep in mind we all will lose a decent amount of muscle initially on this journey, but the hope is to minimize the amount of muscle loss you experience.

Hair loss suggestions: Most people will lose some hair after surgery. The reason you will likely lose some hair after surgery is because your calorie intake is much less. Also because your vitamin stores are needed for other functions in your body when nutrition is less. The best way to minimize hair loss is to make sure you are consistently taking your bariatric vitamins as well as hitting your protein goal. Even if you lose some hair, if you are consistent with these habits, the likelihood of it growing back is much greater. Another piece of advice I have for you when it comes to hair loss is to make sure you aren't over-supplementing. You probably don't need extra hair, skin, nail, and biotin supplements if you are taking your bariatric multivitamins. Your bariatric multi will have everything you need. If you over-supplement, those vitamins might end up competing for absorption, which we don't want. Over-supplementation can also increase the likelihood of hair loss. For example, too much selenium, often found in hair skin and nail vitamins, can actually cause hair loss rather than stopping it.

"What are the best vitamins to take? How do I know what I need? And why do I need to take them for the rest of my life?"

There are many bariatric vitamin brands including Procare, Celebrate, Barilife, Bariatric Advantage, and Bariatric Fusion, to name a few. What's most important is that you are choosing a bariatric-specific vitamin versus an over-the-counter vitamin from your local pharmacy.

Bariatric vitamins are specifically formulated to be better absorbed by bariatric patients and to provide you with the nutrients you need in the proper amounts. Even though bariatric vitamins might cost a bit more, in order to get your needs met, you would zoom through a 30-day supply of over-the-counter or Flintstone vitamins in about two weeks, so they really aren't going to save you much money in the long run.

Making sure you are getting all of your vitamin needs met can feel overwhelming and very time-consuming. In my opinion and experience, the easiest way to make sure you are getting your needs met is to:

- Purchase a bariatric-specific one-a-day multivitamin with iron
- Purchase bariatric-specific 500mg calcium citrate chews (calcium citrate is superior to calcium carbonate for WLS patients due to absorption)

It's important to space out your vitamins by two hours to make sure they are properly absorbed. It's especially important to make sure you are spacing out your calcium from your multivitamin if it has iron or any other iron supplements you may be taking since calcium blocks the absorption of iron. I also suggest taking your multivitamin with food in your stomach. Not only does having food in your stomach increase the absorption of the fat-soluble nutrients (Vitamins A, D, E, and K), but it can also reduce nausea.

Here is a sample vitamin regimen:

- 9:00 a.m.: Breakfast + bariatric one-a-day multivitamin with iron
- 11:00 a.m.: 500mg calcium chew
- 1:00 p.m.: 500mg calcium chew
- 3:00 p.m,: 500 mg calcium chew

Always follow your surgery team's guidelines for vitamin supplementation, and be sure to add in any additional supplements such as additional iron or B12 they may require.

Taking vitamins after weight loss surgery is not optional; it is a lifelong commitment in order to avoid malnutrition. It's definitely one of the less glamorous sides of surgery, but it is necessary.

A common misconception is once you are "far enough post-op," you can stop taking them because you're eating more. Another common misconception is that you don't need to take vitamins long-term if you've had VSG since you don't have malabsorption. Both of these things are false. Even with VSG, it's important to make sure you are taking your vitamins.

Nutrient deficiencies typically won't show up until three or more years post-op. Nutrient deficiencies can lead to some pretty awful outcomes including iron-deficiency anemia and trouble with bone density, including issues with your teeth.

For more resources on vitamins and understanding how much of each vitamin and mineral you need head to www.thesleeveddietitian.com/easy.

"Why can't I count collagen towards my overall daily protein goal?"

Collagen is not a complete protein because it is lacking one of the nine essential amino acids, tryptophan. If you choose to include collagen supplements in your diet, my suggestion is to not count it toward your minimum protein goal for the day. Example: if your goal is 60g of protein and you get 20g of protein from collagen, you really want to aim for 80g for the day to make sure you're not falling short on complete protein.

"Why am I always hungry? I feel like I've been hungry since I had surgery, and I wasn't expecting this."

Everyone's hunger levels are going to be different after surgery. Some people do experience true hunger, even right after surgery. If this is you, don't panic. Being hungry isn't a bad thing, it just means you need to make sure you are eating the foods that are going to fill you up and keep you satisfied. And if you feel like you can't get a handle on your hunger, despite following the bariatric meal plate method and implementing good habits, I would encourage you to speak to your medical team about whether or not you would be a good candidate for a GLP-1 medication in addition to surgery. But please know, if you are hungrier than you thought you would be after surgery, you are not alone and you are not "broken," as many bariatric patients experience this.

"Did I stretch my stomach? Is it possible to stretch your stomach out?"

I see so much panic over stretching your stomach back out after surgery. So here's the deal: your stomach is a muscle. It is going to "stretch" over time. As your internal incisions heal and the inflammation goes down, your stomach will regain some of its elasticity.

However, it is HIGHLY unlikely that you will be able to stretch your stomach out beyond what is expected. While this can happen, it's my understanding that if you have been able to stretch your stomach back out to the point where it is comparable in size to what it was prior to surgery, your surgery itself wasn't performed correctly. Typically, if your surgery was done correctly, this should not happen.

Now, one caveat to this is knowing that if you are continually "pushing" your restriction and eating beyond your fullness levels, over time, you may end up being able to eat more simply because you are not listening to your body and you are pushing it past its limits. This also goes back to that "eating around your restriction" that I talked about in Chapter 7.

If you truly believe your stomach has stretched back out, I would encourage you to reach out to your surgery center so they can do some imaging to see what's going on internally, as this is the only way to know for certain if there is an issue with your pouch.

So the next time you take that one extra bite, or eat more than you think you should, please don't panic. It doesn't mean you are broken or you have stretched out your stomach. And when in doubt, go back to weighing your portions and following the meal plate method. I have a feeling that, if you do, you will start to notice how quickly you get full again.

"What if I've lost too much weight and need to gain weight?"

If you feel you have lost too much weight, make sure you reach out to your bariatric team so they can support you.

If you are looking to gain weight or stop losing weight, you may want to consider trying the "power packing" technique. This is when you increase your calorie intake without increasing the volume of your portions.

This is typically done by using higher fat options. Some examples might be adding peanut butter to shakes or smoothies, using full fat dairy, or cooking with additional oil and butter in order to get more calories in without increasing how much you are eating portion wise.

"Do you have any regrets?"

No, not one, at least not when it comes to having surgery. A lot of people say that their only regret was not doing it sooner, which I can completely understand. I had my surgery at 24 years old, and I'm glad I did. I worry that, had I done it when I was in my teens or earlier twenties, I may not have been ready emotionally or mentally.

If I regret anything though, I regret waiting until I started to lose weight to believe in myself and allow myself to be happy. I wish I hadn't allowed myself to sit on the sidelines of my own life for so long. I wish I hadn't missed out on so many experiences because of my weight. I wish I had realized then how damn capable I was.

This might sound corny, but this journey reminds me of *The Wizard of Oz.* Dorothy had the ruby slippers the whole time; she never needed anything she didn't already have to take her home.

Each and every one of us is capable of believing in ourselves every step of the way on this journey. I wish I had realized that sooner. And while I didn't have everything I needed to overcome my struggles, both with my weight and self-esteem, because I truly needed this surgery to save me, I did have the ability to be kinder to myself and allow myself to be happy despite the number on the scale.

"What's been your favorite non-scale victory?"

The NSVs (non-scale victories, meaning, the wins you experience that aren't related to the number on the scale) are by far my favorite parts of this journey. And my goodness, do I have so many.

But I think I experience my favorite NSVs when I travel and when I go to Disney World. (It's my happy place.) It's so near and dear to my heart, and being able to go, in the body I have now, is something I will never take for granted.

It's still amazing to me to be able to walk through the airport, not out of breath or sweating as I try to lug my suitcase around. Being able to fit in an airplane seat and not need a seatbelt extender will just never get old, nor will being able to fit on all the rides and not worry about being escorted off because of my size. It's also SO incredible to walk miles and miles all day in the heat without constantly having to stop and take breaks. It's also so freeing to me to have a vacation where I'm not hyperfocused or fixated on all the food and all the Disney snacks and Disney treats. They are simply part of the experience, not the whole experience. And to be able to go into any Disney merch store and buy myself a any T-shirt or sweatshirt I want is something I know some people may never bat an eye at, but for me and for anyone who knows how hard it is to find clothes when you are bigger, it means the absolute world to be able to choose a hoodie I adore versus resorting to what is left that will fit or walking out empty-handed.

As wonderful as it is when you hit a new milestone on the scale, NOTHING could possibly feel as good as the NSVs. So remember, it is NOT all about the scale, it is about so much more than that. It's about being healthy and happy enough to live the fulfilling life you always imagined for yourself.

"What's your best piece of advice for someone on a bariatric journey? What do you wish you knew before you had surgery?"

This might be my favorite question to answer. *So I'm going to give you my top five tips and things I wish I knew when I first started my journey.*

1. *Fall in love with the process, not the destination*

Don't wait until you hit a number on the scale to be happy. If you do, I worry you will be disappointed. Not because you will be disappointed in your weight loss, but because you might be disappointed in how you feel when it's not the fireworks and balloons you were hoping for.

And in order to make everything you are working for become sustainable long-term, you can't be miserable and "white-knuckling it" every day. Sure, some days will be hard, and it's not all rainbows and butterflies, but you need to figure out how to enjoy your day-to-day routine to make it a lifestyle, not a temporary fix.

2. *Choose an exercise you would do every day, even if it never resulted in weight loss.*

I really can't stress this one enough. So many people only exercise or add movement to their routine for the purpose of weight loss. And far too many people use exercise as a form of punishment for something they ate.

Moving your body consistently is so important. Not only does it help you burn calories for weight loss, but it helps you maintain muscle mass on your body. When you do that, your BMR (basal metabolic rate, i.e., the calories you burn at rest) will be higher. When your BMR is higher, you are able to sustain eating more calories as time goes on. Not to mention it is so good for your emotional and mental health as well as your physical health.

I never thought I would fall in love with working out, but here I am three years into joining my local CrossFit gym, and I absolutely love it. I go because I want to. Because it feels good. Because I enjoy the community aspect. And I keep going back for all those non-scale-related benefits.

I tell everyone to try as many different types of exercises as you can to see what you do and don't like. Try yoga, Pilates, Orange Theory, Zumba, etc.—so many things to try! You won't know what you just might fall in love with until you put yourself out there and try new things.

3. *Get support and work on your mindset; you probably need it more than you realize.*

I think it's really hard to admit that you need and deserve help and support on this journey. Working on your mindset and your emotional well-being on this journey is so crucial. No one should be doing this all alone. Head to chapters 12 and 17 to learn more about how to work on your mindset and finding your community and support system on this journey.

4. *Stop using the scale as your only measure of success (and happiness).*

Just because the scale isn't moving doesn't mean you aren't progressing. Instead of only tracking your weight, also keep track of your measurements, how you are sleeping, your mood, and your activity level.

I highly recommend only getting on the scale MAX one time per week. So often I see people running to the scale every day, sometimes even multiple times per day. If the scale goes down, they use it as a way to validate their hard work and allow themselves to feel good and be happy. But if it goes up, they use it as a way to berate or punish themselves. Please don't do that. The number doesn't tell the whole picture. Focus more on how you are feeling and your habits and less on the number itself.

5. *Don't make it harder than it has to be.*

This journey is hard, that's for sure. There's nothing about this that's "easy." But so often, I see people wayyyyy overthinking and way overcomplicating things. It does not have to be excruciating in order for you to be "successful."

Follow your post-op guidelines. Don't try to bend the rules or find loopholes. Go by your plan and add foods as you're able to. Eat foods you actually like that are on your plan and continue to add to your plate as you're ready. Move your body more days than you are sedentary. Focus on your water and your vitamins and check those two non-negotiables off every day. And get support and work on your mindset.

I promise, it doesn't have to be more complicated than that. Overthinking and worrying only is going to stress you out, deter you, and potentially lead to self-sabotage. Take it day by day, moment by moment, meal by meal.

You got this. Even when things feel uncertain and even when you hit bumps in the road. Sometimes on this journey there will be setbacks, and even complications, but I promise if you are faced with those hurdles, there are ways to overcome them too.

Bite-Sized Recap

- There's no right or wrong way to navigate post-surgery life.
- Be mindful of who you take advice from on this journey, specifically pertaining to nutrition and medical advice.
- Remember, the advice I give you here is based on my own experiences as both a professional and patient, but that doesn't mean everything I suggest is going to work for you. I encourage you to take these tidbits of advice and apply what feels right for you to your own routine.
- It's also important to remember what worked for one person might not work for everyone.
- Fall in love with the process, not just the destination.
- Try not to overcomplicate things. This journey is definitely hard, but it doesn't need to be overwhelming every step of the way.

For journal prompts and resources related to this chapter be sure to head to www.thesleeveddietitian.com/easy.

Chapter 11
Sometimes It's Complicated: Regain & Complications After WLS

com·pli·cat·ed

/kämpləkādəd/

adjective

1. consisting of many interconnecting parts or elements; intricate

"a complicated situation to be in"

2. Medicine, involving complications

"complicated gastrointestinal issues after surgery"

It's Not All Sunshine and Rainbows

Even though weight loss surgery is the gold standard for treating obesity and is considered a very safe and low-risk procedure, just like with any surgery, there are risks associated. And just like every other weight loss intervention and treatment, it is not perfect. I'd be doing you all a disservice if I didn't discuss some of the potential risks, outcomes, and complications of weight loss surgery.

Regain

When I first had my weight loss surgery, I'll admit I was ignorant to the realities of regain. While I knew most people don't stay at their lowest weight, and that some rebound weight was normal, I didn't realize regain was a reality for so many people.

I swore that would never be me. And I must admit, I shake my head at the 2018, newly post-op version of Jamie. My naive brain, at the time, was even a bit judgmental. I used to think, *Oh, that will never be me. I can't imagine going through all of this just to put myself back in that position. All you have to do is stick to your habits, and you'll be fine. Clearly people who are regaining their weight aren't doing what they are supposed to.*

And in that moment, I believe the universe was listening in and decided, *"Touché. Let's humble her real quick."*

I want you to read very closely. I'm going to tell you what I wish I had known all those years ago: no one is immune to regain. No one is better than anyone else on this journey. And no one should be judging anyone else for regaining their weight. Because remember, obesity is a disease, not a moral failing. And I suppose that younger version of myself still didn't quite grasp that.

Certainly, habits play a large part in maintaining your weight loss, but there are other factors as well. Set point theory is real and not only occurs in those pre-WLS, but also those post WLS. Obesity is a chronic disease, which means even once you've lost weight, you will still have to manage all of your habits and the symptoms that come along with obesity.

I hit my then lowest weight at about 9 or 10 months post-op. Even though I didn't want to stop losing weight at that point, I did. From there, I went on to maintain a range within 5–10 lbs. or so of that weight for nearly two years. And I was okay with that. Until year three post-op rolled around. God, did I struggle.

As I shared earlier, in August of 2020, I had my IUD removed, which I truly feel contributed to my onset of struggles with regain after having maintained it for so long.

I had it placed long before my VSG, and even though it was *supposed* to be nonhormonal, I'll be damned if that didn't royally mess up my hormones. After its removal, I shot up 15 pounds over the course of a month. In addition to that quick regain, for the first time since I had had my weight loss surgery, I had noticed PCOS symptoms that had since been in remission resurfacing, including acne, thinning hair, and fatigue. In that same month, I had also joined CrossFit, and while some muscle gain may have been happening, that 15 pounds was certainly not completely muscle. And other than that, nothing changed in my routine. I wasn't eating more. I wasn't deviating from my habits, and I really didn't feel like I was "slacking" in any way.

The reason I share these circumstances in great detail is because whenever someone is struggling with regain, they are almost immediately met with accusations of them not "trying hard enough" or assumptions that they've "fallen off the wagon." Sometimes, yes, habits do slip, and that absolutely plays a role. But with good old obesity and all its complexities, we know that there are factors beyond just willpower and lifestyle that contribute to weight gain. Hormones, amongst other factors, play such huge roles in our bodies' overall functioning.

Sometimes there are factors that are beyond our control. So if you've been struggling or have struggled with regain, and you've thought "but I'm doing all I can," while feeling like people around you didn't believe that you were doing all you could, I want you to know that I believe you. I see you. I was there too.

So I was back to white-knuckling it again. And I did what I knew I should do: I scheduled an appointment with my surgery center. I knew that if I was struggling, they would be the best place for me to go for support and to see what was going on. Right? Theoretically, yes. But that wasn't the case.

My surgeon all but nearly refused to see me. She had the receptionist relay a message to me over the phone: "Doctor X wanted to make sure you understood before you take the time to come in that she will not prescribe any medications to you, and the only option is a revision surgery; otherwise, she can't help."

I was so mad and so insulted. Not only was I offended that she thought I was just coming in for medication (and at the time, GLP-1s weren't even on my radar), but also that she just didn't want to help me.

Despite my better judgment, I went in for the appointment. She pretty much told me that I was "doing everything right" and that I had still exceeded her expectations for me, so I should be "fine." But I wasn't fine. I was not okay with such rapid gain happening so quickly for what felt like no reason.

My surgeon had me sit down with their new dietitian on staff, one who I had never met before and who had no idea I was a dietitian too. But I wasn't opposed to meeting her. For all I knew, maybe there was something in my habits I was overlooking.

So I sat down with her, and she did what's called a "dietary recall," which is where a dietitian asks a patient to recount everything they eat throughout a typical day. She really had no feedback for me, at least none that was useful. The only thing she decided to focus on was my afternoon snack of cashews and fruit. She proceeded to pull out a ¼ cup measuring cup from her desk drawer to "make sure I knew what an actual ¼ cup looked like" so I wasn't "overeating them." It took a lot of restraint for me not to slam her door on the way out.

At that moment, I realized how unhelpful so many WLS centers are when it comes to regain. I had never been so insulted in my life. The way she tried to belittle me by insinuating I didn't know what a ¼ cup serving looked like was just wild. She didn't need to know I was a dietitian. She shouldn't have been speaking to anyone as if they were incompetent, or making them feel like they must be overeating or doing something "wrong."

Throughout that entire next year, I continued to struggle. I felt like I was "white-knuckling it" again. I felt like weight loss was so excruciatingly hard. And I also noticed my PCOS symptoms coming back with a vengeance. Things

I hadn't struggled with in years became a reality again: missed and irregular periods, acne, and immense struggles with the scale despite every effort to keep the weight off.

By summer of 2022, even though I had still been following the meal plate method, working out consistently, and sticking to all the "good" habits I had worked so hard to create over the years, the scale was up 28 pounds from my lowest. And while that was not the worst-case scenario, I just couldn't sit there any longer and watch the scale continue to climb.

That's when I reached out to Dr. Spencer Nadolsky, an obesity specialist physician I looked up to and admired, to see if he and his medical weight loss program, Sequence, could help me. From there, I went on Mounjaro, which has truly been game-changing for me. Since then, after regaining 28 lbs, I have lost 40 lbs. and hit a new adult low weight. And to be honest? I feel healthier than ever before. Not just because I tackled the weight or because I got my PCOS symptoms back under control, but because now I'm able to reap the benefits of all the habits I've been working so hard to stick with.

And I'm SO glad that, despite every moment of that year and half I spent struggling, I kept going. I kept going to CrossFit; I kept planning my meals; I kept getting my protein and fiber in. And now I'm even healthier than the first time I lost weight, because I have been able to sustain so much muscle mass on my body, and I truly feel stronger than ever.

I want you to know that if you are struggling with regain and feel like you have been doing everything within your power to keep the weight off and lose it, I believe you. I believe you when you say you are trying and doing your best and just don't understand why the weight is coming back on or why the things you were doing before aren't working now.

And if you are early on in your journey, or you are pre-op, I'm not sharing any of this to scare you. I just want you to know that regain is a possibility. And even though we may be far better off with a little regain post-op than we were before surgery, it is valid to not want to struggle with it.

And I'd be lying to you if I promised that good habits alone will solve all your problems. The habits are SO important, that's for sure. But there are other things there too: hormonal factors, biological factors, genetic factors, emotional factors, and environmental factors. And you deserve help in tackling regain, no matter which of those factors you are struggling with. Because weight struggles are not a moral failing, and you are not a failure because you regained.

How to Tackle Regain from a Habit Perspective: The Things That Are within Your Control

If you are struggling with regain, it's important to first take a look at your habits and routines. It's important to take ownership over the parts of your journey that you do have control over. I've made some suggestions below. But please note that, in addition to these suggestions, it's also important to work alongside a registered dietitian who is encouraging and supportive (you might have to "shop" around for one until you find one you jibe with) and seek emotional support in a therapist, psychiatrist, and/or support group to address any underlying issues.

Now, when it comes to refining your habits to start to tackle regain, I have a three-step method I use with my clients: Reflect, Acknowledge, Plan & Implement.

Below I give you an overview of this process for tackling regain, however, if you would like a more in-depth guide through this process, please visit www.thesleeveddietitian.com/easy for additional worksheets and materials.

Reflect

When you're struggling with regain, it's REALLY tempting to jump headfirst into a diet or strict routine.

Instead, I would like to challenge you to reflect. Take a look back at your journey as a whole before changing anything. What things were you doing at the beginning of your journey that perhaps you are not doing now? (And I don't mean just eating smaller portions—increasing portion sizes is a given.)

What habits were you continually doing each and every day when you were losing weight that perhaps you are not doing now? What events led to where you are now?

If you could look back and change one thing, what would it be? What, specifically, would you change?

Spend some time truly reflecting on the questions above before you attempt to tackle the regain or make any changes.

Acknowledge

Once you've spent some time reflecting on your journey, which pieces can you acknowledge that you have the power to change?

It's easy to make excuses. Life gets hard, things happen, and we are faced with challenges. But of the overwhelming struggles you have faced or are facing right now, which do you have control over?

We can't control what happens in the world around us, but we CAN control how we respond to things. I'd like you to take some time to own up, acknowledge, and admit the things you have the ability to change. This piece can be especially difficult. Being honest with ourselves can be challenging, but once we can acknowledge what we can do, we can then make a game plan.

I would like for you to acknowledge the specific habits that may have contributed to regain.

Plan & Implement

Once you are able to zoom out and acknowledge some things you could work on improving or changing, I suggest coming up with a plan in order to make those changes in a sustainable and realistic way.

If there are lots of things on your acknowledgment list, that is OKAY! I don't want you to feel overwhelmed or like you have to tackle all these things at once. In fact, that's the last thing I want you to do.

I want you to start working at the things on your list slowly.

How to Tackle Regain from a Medical Perspective

Nutrition and lifestyle habits will always be a part of your bariatric journey. You cannot tackle obesity and manage it without those pieces.

However, if you have been working on your habits and are still feeling stuck, you might want to consider speaking with your medical or surgical team about alternative options.

Medications

AOMs (anti-obesity medications) might be an important tool for you as you start to tackle your regain. I strongly encourage you to speak with your surgical team to see if you might be a good candidate for an AOM. And if your surgical team is not in support of AOM usage, first send them my book to read, then go find another surgeon or obesity specialist physician who stays up-to-date on evidence-based research for obesity treatment. Because you deserve a comprehensive bariatric treatment plan if you are struggling with regain. (Head back to Chapters 4 and 5 for more information on AOMs, or head to www.thesleeveddietitian.com/easy for more resources on how to find double board-certified physicians and resources on medication management.)

Revision Surgeries

In some cases of regain, you may be a candidate for a revision surgery. A revision surgery is when they either "redo" your weight loss surgery or convert one surgery type to another (for example: lap band to VSG or VSG to RNY or DS).

There isn't a standard cutoff or qualification to meet to qualify for a revision surgery, and this is something that should be assessed on an individual basis with your surgical team. Keep in mind that only those with "substantial" amounts of regain are eligible. Revision surgeries can also be performed due to complications.

Additionally, it's important to keep in mind that revision surgeries for regain don't typically result in as much weight loss as your initial surgery. And in order to qualify for a revision surgery and to have insurance pay for it in the US, you likely will have to redo the 3–6 month pre-op process.

In some cases, revision surgeries are planned ahead of time. These are called "staged" surgeries. One of the most common staged procedures is the VSG to DS surgery. Some patients, particularly those starting at very high BMIs, will begin with a VSG; then, once they hit a certain weight loss goal or benchmark set by their surgeon, they will do a second WLS, such as the DS. The reason they may do this is so the patient can achieve optimal weight loss. Doing this can also make their initial surgery safer, since they wouldn't have to be under anesthesia as long.

Regardless of your reason for having a revision surgery, know you are not a failure, and having a WLS revision isn't shameful. If having a revision is going to help you overcome obesity and be the happiest and healthiest version of you, then it is absolutely the best option for you and your journey.

Complications

Complications after weight loss surgery are not as common as one might assume. According to the ASMBS, "The risk of death associated with bariatric surgery is about 0.1% and the overall likelihood of major complications is about 4%."[97] To give you a frame of reference, weight loss surgery is about as risky as having your appendix removed. Statistically speaking, having a hip replacement is a far riskier procedure.

However, that's not to say that complications do not occur at all. Minor and short-term complications can happen, as well as more serious and long-term complications. When it comes to having weight loss surgery, your medical team will determine if you are at risk for any of these complications. And remember, the benefits of WLS must far outweigh the potential complications in order for you to qualify for surgery. The majority of the most common complications listed below are easily treatable.

Potential Early Post-Surgical Complications

Potential Complication	What That Means	Prevention/ Treatment
Leaks	Digestive secretions from the stomach leak out of a hole or seam in the new stomach or pouch. RNY and VSG leaks are different. A VSG leak is considered more difficult to treat and occurs in 1–7% of VSG patients. Leaks are most likely to occur within three days after surgery.	Post-op patients who display signs and symptoms of tachycardia or hypotension should be evaluated for potential leak. Patients who present with leaks likely will need to have it surgically repaired.

[97] ASMBS, "U.S. Obesity Rate Higher Than Ever."

Stenosis, twists, stricture, and kinks	Food or liquids are not able to pass through from the esophagus to the pouch or new stomach. RNY stenosis is common, occurring in 8–19% of RNY patients, and is easy to diagnose and often treatable without another operation. It is less likely to occur in VSG patients, affecting approximately 1–2% of patients.	Dilation is performed to open up the diameter of where the stenosis/stricture is. It can take as many as three dilations before the patient can eat comfortably. This often can be done nonsurgically.
Bleeding	Post-op bleeding that requires medical intervention occurs in up to 11% of both RNY and VSG patients. The staple line/surgical site is the most common site of bleeding.	Patients with a history of dysmetabolic syndrome have a higher risk of excessive post-op bleeding. Fortunately, 85% of patients are likely to stop bleeding without surgical intervention or further treatment. Therapeutic interventions such as clips or epinephrine injections are the first line of treatment.
Venous thromboembolism (VTE) (also known as a blood clot)	The rate of a VTE after WLS is very low. However, a pulmonary embolism (PE) is the most common cause of mortality after WLS procedures.	Those with a BMI >50, those whose surgery is anticipated to be >4 hours, patients with hypercoagulable states, and those with hypoventilation syndrome are at greater risk for VTE and PE. Losing weight prior to surgery, stopping birth control pills or medications that may lead to blood clots, and taking heparin injections post-op can help prevent a VTE and PE.

Nausea/vomiting	Some nausea and vomiting is normal and anticipated as part of the recovery process post-op. This may also occur as a result of pain medications and/or anesthesia from surgery.	Usually, nausea and vomiting resolves over time. Be sure to follow post-op diet instructions and stay hydrated by taking small sips of fluid often. You may also be prescribed antiemetics such as Zofran. If it persists long term, be sure to let your team know to ensure there are no other underlying issues and/or issues with getting your nutritional needs met.

Sources: Robert Lim et al., "Early and Late Complications of Bariatric Operation," *Trauma Surgery and Acute Care Open* 3, no. 1 (2018), https://tsaco.bmj.com/content/3/1/e000219; "Bariatric Surgery Risks, Complications, and Side Effects," Weight Loss Services, University of Pittsburgh Medical Center, https://www.upmc.com/services/bariatrics/candidate/risks-and-complications.

Potential Long-Term Complications Post Surgery

Potential Complication	What That Means	Prevention/Treatment
Band slippage	This only occurs in gastric banding/lap band patients. This is when one wall, or side of the stomach, slips through the orifice of the band, resulting in a larger-than-normal gastric pouch superior to the band. It's considered the most common post-op gastric band complication, occurring in 8% of patients.	Fundoplication around the band and the *pars flaccida* technique for placement of the band are thought to reduce the likelihood of band slippage. Technical precautions should be taken by your surgeon during the time of the band placement. Signs and symptoms of a slipped band may include vomiting after meals, fullness only relieved by vomiting, and pain/irritation of the upper abdomen. The first line of treatment is to completely empty the band fluid. Band removal may be performed. Many lap band patients will convert to VSG in this case.

Acid reflux/ GERD (also known as heartburn)	Acid reflux/GERD is most common in VSG patients. This is when stomach acid or bile flows back up into your esophagus. Approximately 35% of VSG patients may experience new or worsened reflux. Regaining weight after surgery may potentially worsen acid reflux symptoms.	Acid reflux may be managed with dietary and lifestyle changes such as limiting highly acidic foods, caffeine, and refined carbohydrates. Sitting upright after meals and avoiding large meals, especially at night, may be helpful. Some patients may need medications, such as proton pump inhibitors (PPIs), to manage reflux. In more severe cases, some may undergo a minimally invasive procedure known as the LINX or convert to a gastric bypass.
Constipation	Constipation is common and may occur after surgery. This is often from a decrease in food intake as well as a decrease in fiber. Typically, constipation goes away with time once you are able to eat and drink more.	Be sure to increase your fluids and make sure you are getting adequate hydration. With the guidance of your bariatric team, you may also need to incorporate fiber supplements and/or laxatives.
Gallstones/ gallbladder issues	Those who have WLS are at a higher risk of developing gallstones compared to the rest of the population due to hormonal changes and increased cholesterol saturation of gallbladder bile due to weight loss.	Limiting dietary fat and consuming high-fiber carbohydrates may help reduce your risk of gallstones. In some cases, your surgeon may put you on a medication to help reduce your risk of gallstones. Approximately 15% of bariatric patients will require a cholecystectomy (gallbladder removal).
Perforation	Spontaneous gastric perforation (a hole that develops through the wall of a body organ) occurs in 1–2% of bariatric patients, some without warning signs. Untreated gastric ulcers may lead to a perforation.	Avoid NSAIDs (anti-inflammatory drugs) and tobacco use/ smoking. The treatment for this is surgery, either laparoscopic or open, to repair the perforation.

Gastric ulcers	A gastric ulcer is a sore that develops on the lining of the esophagus, stomach, or small intestine. Common causes include the bacteria H. pylori and use of NSAIDs. Gastric ulcers may also be called "marginal ulcers," and they can occur around or near your incision line. Signs and symptoms include upper abdominal pain, bloating, gas, vomiting, and loss of appetite.	Avoiding smoking and NSAIDs can help reduce your risk for ulcers. It's also suggested to avoid alcohol and foods that cause you discomfort. Managing stress levels may also reduce your risk of ulcers. Various medications are used to treat ulcers, and in some cases, surgical treatment may be necessary.
Small bowel obstruction	A small bowel obstruction is a blockage in the small intestine, most often caused by scar tissue (often from prior surgeries where the tissue forms adhesions) or a hernia in bariatric patients.	Signs and symptoms include abdominal pain, bloating, distension, nausea, and vomiting. More than 50% of small bowel obstructions in bariatric patients are due to internal hernias. Treatments may include fluids, bowel rest, antiemetics for nausea, bowel decompression through a nasogastric tube, or surgery.
Internal hernia	An internal hernia (IH) is defined as the protrusion of abdominal viscera, most commonly small bowel loops, through a peritoneal or mesenteric aperture into a compartment in the abdominal and pelvic cavity. Although uncommon, this would be considered a more severe complication that can occur in post RNY patients, especially those who had small bowel obstruction symptoms.	Typically, 70% of internal hernias can be corrected laparoscopically, but may also need to be converted to an open operation if needed.

Reactive hypoglycemia	This is a low-blood-sugar episode that occurs after a meal, typically 1–4 hours after. This is most common after RNY, but it may occur after other bariatric procedures as well. Symptoms of reactive hypoglycemia include shakiness, dizziness, anxiety, sweating, rapid heart rate, fatigue, and hunger.	You may have to monitor your blood sugar to ensure your sugars do not drop too low. Ideally, you want your sugars at 70 mg/dL or less. In order to bring your blood sugar up, it is recommended to consume 15 grams of simple carbohydrates at a time until your sugars have increased. Eating smaller, more frequent meals paired with protein and fats may help. You should work with your bariatric team to see what regimen is best for you.
Vitamin deficiencies, macronutrient deficiencies, and malnutrition	All bariatric patients are susceptible to micro and macronutrient deficiencies after WLS, which may lead to clinical malnutrition. This is due to lowered dietary intake as well as anatomical alterations to the GI tract, where vitamins and nutrients are often absorbed. Those who undergo non-malabsorptive procedures are susceptible to nutrient deficiencies (iron, B12, calcium, and protein deficiencies are most common).	Most nutrient deficiencies can be prevented with proper vitamin and protein supplementation and lifelong nutritional monitoring via bloodwork.

Sources: Robert Lim et al., "Early and Late Complications of Bariatric Operation," *Trauma Surgery and Acute Care Open* 3, no. 1 (2018), https://tsaco.bmj.com/content/3/1/e000219; "Bariatric Surgery Risks, Complications, and Side Effects," Weight Loss Services, University of Pittsburgh Medical Center, https://www.upmc.com/services/bariatrics/candidate/risks-and-complications; "What We Know about Reflux After Gastric Sleeve," Surgical Association of Mobile, P.A. website, accessed on July 14, 2023, https://sampadocs.com/2019/12/23/reflux-after-gastric-sleeve/; Victor B. Tsirline, "How Frequently and When Do Patients Undergo Cholecystectomy after Bariatric Surgery?," *Surgery for Obesity and Related Diseases* 10, no. 2 (March–April 2014): 313–321, https://pubmed.ncbi.nlm.nih.gov/24462305/; Marina Lanzetta Monica et al., "Internal Hernias: A Difficult Diagnostic Challenge. Review of CT Signals and Clinical Findings," *Acta Biomedica* 90, no. 5: 20–37, https://www.ncbi.nlm.nih.gov/pmc/articles/PMC6625567/; Roberta Lupoli, "Bariatric Surgery and Long-Term Nutritional Issues," *World Journal of Diabetes* 8, no. 11 (November 2017): 464–474, https://www.ncbi.nlm.nih.gov/pmc/articles/PMC5700383/.

Remember, the benefits of surgery must outweigh the potential risks of any of the above complications, which is why it's so important to undergo all of the pre-op testing and counseling prior to surgery so you can understand the potential risks and discuss the best surgical options with your team.

Bite-Sized Recap

- Even though weight loss surgery is the gold standard for treating obesity and is considered a very safe and low-risk procedure, as with any surgery, there are risks associated.
- Regaining weight post-op is a struggle many surgical weight loss patients will face at some point in their journey. While it is normal to fluctuate, and it's normal to not stay at your lowest weight forever, it can also feel really defeating to struggle with regain.
- It is possible to tackle regain both through evaluating and modifying habits, as well as using additional tools such as anti-obesity medications and/or revision surgeries.
- Minor and short-term complications can happen, as well as more serious and long-term complications, after weight loss surgery. When it comes to having weight loss surgery, your medical team will determine if you are at risk for any of these complications. And remember, the benefits of WLS must far outweigh the potential complications in order for you to qualify for surgery.

For journal prompts and resources related to this chapter be sure to head to www.thesleeveddietitian.com/easy.

Chapter 12
Eww, Feelings

feel·ings

fēliNG/

noun; plural noun: feelings

1. an emotional state or reaction

"a feeling of joy"

2. a belief, especially a vague or irrational one

"She had the feeling that she was always going to struggle."

Reminder

I'd like to preface this chapter by reminding you that I am not a therapist or licensed mental health professional. In this chapter, I'm simply sharing my personal opinion, as well as discussing the feelings and emotions I've seen others express on this journey.

This chapter also discusses my approach to mindfulness and awareness after surgery, from a bariatric coaching perspective; however, please keep in mind you should always discuss your mindset practices with your own therapist or mental healthcare provider.

Getting into Our Feelings

In my membership program, T.R.I.B.E.®, one of our ongoing running inside jokes is "ewwww, feelings." During our support groups, we talk a lot about our feelings and emotions—it's truly one of the only ways to figure out what's going on in our journey. Whether that be feeling stuck, overwhelmed, worried, or just generally self-sabotaging, we are never going to be able to overcome those struggles if we don't recognize what it is that's truly going on. But feelings make us uncomfortable, which is why we so readily stuffed them down our whole lives. Hence the joke "ewww, feelings" anytime we're encouraged to talk about them.

And I'll tell you what I tell my clients and members: *you cannot solve an emotional problem with a nutritional solution.*

I know, I was disappointed to learn that one too. But I hate to break it to you: you're not going to solve your problems, your emotional eating, or your self-sabotaging behaviors, by me throwing a diet plan or calorie goal at you.

I wish someone had told me just how important it is to work on your mindset on this journey. It's true—we have surgery on our stomachs, not our heads.

I think, logically, I understood this going into surgery, but I didn't truly "get it" until I was in it. I really believe this aspect is what makes weight loss surgery so hard.

Even though I had a long history of disordered eating patterns (which I'll dive into a bit later), I still didn't identify as an emotional eater. I simply didn't realize I was one. That was, until I wasn't able to actually engage in emotional eating.

During my two-week liquid pre-op diet, I truly recognized how much of an emotional eater I was for the first time. Those two weeks were HARD. For me, that was one of the hardest parts of my whole journey.

I started my pre-op liquid diet on December 5, 2017, and I wasn't cleared to progress onto pureed foods until nearly three weeks post-op, on January 5. It was a full five weeks on liquids. And especially during the holiday season, this brought up so many emotions.

You know what I did during those five weeks? I cried. Every. Single. Day. And let me just say, as a Capricorn and Enneagram 8, I'm NOT a crier (which, perhaps, maybe that's my problem?), so this was alarming.

I wasn't crying because the hunger pains were unbearable. I mean yes, liquids aren't exactly filling, but the protein shakes did their job. What I realized was, in those moments when I was stressed, overwhelmed, anxious, bored, etc., and I wanted to soothe myself with food but couldn't, I was left not knowing what to do. I literally had no idea how to process everything I was feeling without food.

At the time, I felt like the pre-op diet was so cruel. But after, looking back, even though it was really challenging, I'm really grateful I had to go through that. It was the first time I realized how much mindset work I had ahead of me.

And the mindset challenges haven't stopped since then. This whole journey is one big mind f*ck. Whether that's struggling with body image, changing habits, learning to cope, or processing emotions, it all starts with our mindset. Unfortunately, you can't bypass the emotional work (no pun intended). Acknowledging your feelings and your own emotions is truly the first step to changing your mindset, your behaviors, and overcoming emotional eating. Because we cannot change what we don't acknowledge.

The Feelings That Keep Us Stuck

After working with hundreds of people on their bariatric journeys, I've noticed some recurring themes when it comes to emotions. There seems to be a core set of emotions that keeps people stuck, whether that's them putting off surgery and getting help, taking the plunge, or not progressing once they have surgery.

Emotions That Often Keep People from Moving Forward with Surgery

Pride & Ego	For a lot of people, it's really hard to swallow their pride or put their egos aside in order to ask for help or realize they need help beyond just diet and exercise.
Shame & Guilt	Admitting they need help or "can't" do it "on their own" without surgery can bring up a lot of shame and guilt. It can feel very shameful to need to go to a "last resort" or to admit "defeat."
Fear	Fear is a big one. A lot of people are afraid of surgery and fear of the unknown. Some of the most common fears I see include the following: Fear of change Fear of loose skin Fear of hair falling out Fear of partners leaving them Fear of gaining it all back Fear of complications Fear of death

There are, of course, other emotions that keep people from moving forward with surgery, but these seem to be the biggest ones that I see. And I just want to take a moment to say that ANYTHING you feel on this journey, whether before or after, is completely valid and justified. If you are scared of being left with loose skin, or if you are fearful of your hair falling out, that's valid. It's not silly. And it's something that you need to work through *before* you take the plunge.

Emotions That Often Keep People from Hitting Their Goals After Surgery

Anger & Frustration	Anger is something I notice a lot after surgery. So many people express to me that they are angry and frustrated that, despite every change they've made, they still struggle. Or they express they are angry and resentful that they still spend so much time and energy worrying and thinking about food and their bodies. Some are angry to realize that even after surgery, obesity is going to be a lifelong battle.
Overwhelm & Confusion	A lot of people struggle with feeling overwhelmed and confused with what's "right" or what's considered "good" on this journey. There are a LOT of habits to manage and changes to make, and that is very overwhelming and certainly confusing when you don't have support or clear guidance.
Loneliness	Many feel lonely and feel like no one understands them or "gets it," especially if no one else in their life has ever gone through weight loss surgery.
Sadness & Grief	Mourning your "old life" or old lifestyle can bring about a lot of grief and sadness. It's not silly to miss food or to miss your old coping mechanisms. It's a very valid experience.
Inferiority & Unworthiness	So many struggle to see their worth. I see so many people who feel like they don't deserve the success they are experiencing. And there are also those who feel like nothing they ever do is "good enough."

Doubt & Fear	Just like before surgery, fear is a big emotion after too. So many people doubt and fear whether or not this is "too good to be true," or they fear regain.

These feelings are very real and common to experience. I think it's important to actually allow ourselves to feel and recognize them versus pushing them down or to the side.

What I see happening for a lot of people is they don't know how to express or cope with these feelings, which further causes overwhelm and ends up contributing to self-sabotaging behaviors. It makes them feel like they are never going to hit their goals or be "successful."

And while all your experiences are very real and valid, I'd also like to point out that some of these worries and fears are further feeding your **limiting beliefs**. Limiting beliefs are things we tell ourselves are true, when in actuality, they are just lies and false narratives we feed ourselves in order to protect ourselves and keep us safe. And I'd like to share with you how I've worked to overcome these challenges myself.

My Mindset Evolution

One of the things that I've learned about mindset work is that it's kind of like pulling back the layers of an onion. Mindset work is a never-ending journey in itself once you start it.

I didn't really start working on my mindset in a strategic way until the beginning of 2020, a little over two years into my weight loss surgery journey and right at the start of the pandemic.

I had been in therapy for years, but for some reason, "mindset" work feels different to me than "therapy." I recently saw a quote that said, "Therapy is there to help you identify the problem, and mindset work is meant to help you work through it and overcome it." I'm not sure who to credit that quote to, or how true that is (and I realize therapy helps you work through problems as well), but somehow, this made sense to me.

I'm a firm believer that everyone should work with a therapist on this journey AND practice mindset work and practices daily.

At the start of 2020, I started working with my first ever coach. I had hired a business coach to help me take my nutrition coaching business from a "side hustle" to a career I could support myself with.

What I realized in working with her was that I had a lot of major roadblocks, doubts, and limiting beliefs that had nothing to do with my weight, but with how I thought about myself. These roadblocks kept me stuck and kept me from taking action.

During this time, it truly was "sink or swim" in terms of getting my business off the ground. I signed on to work with my business coach at the end of February 2020; I had just gotten married on February 1; and on March 11, I had my first round of plastic surgery for excess skin removal after my weight loss. I ended up having the last elective surgery at my local hospital, where my surgery was performed; and on March 13, the state of Connecticut was shut down.

Timing was on my side, because I had six weeks of medical leave approved for my surgery recovery, which meant I didn't have to work during this time.. During that time, I started implementing everything my business coach was teaching me. Not only did I want nothing more than to get to work with bariatric patients full time in my own business, but I also viewed it as a "now or never" situation. Up until this point, I had been working in a long-term care facility that had already been draining my energy and passion for nutrition. Adding the first ever global pandemic on top of it? I knew it wasn't something I wanted to run back to. (Shoutout to all our healthcare heroes who didn't have a choice in the matter. I want you to know you are loved and appreciated for everything you sacrificed.)

The reason I share this with you is because my business coach didn't just share business strategies with me. No, before she even gave me one single business tip, she had me working on my mindset. It seemed funny and odd, but hey, I was willing to try anything.

So I spent those first six weeks of the pandemic journaling every single morning. She had me working on gratitude, doing affirmations, and working through limiting beliefs. She also gave me journal prompts and hard questions to ask myself.

It felt funny. And as I wrote the affirmations down, I felt like a complete and total impostor. I felt like I didn't "buy" into it. (And I didn't.) But I was willing to go along with it. I mean, heck, I was paying someone to help me, so the least I could do was follow the things they said, right? It was really the first time I'd ever stopped and paused long enough to ask myself how I was truly feeling and to have honest conversations with myself about my wants, needs, desires, and goals.

You wanna know what's funny? It's been over three years, and I still to this day follow that same mindset routine religiously. Not because I have to, but because I genuinely feel better when I do. And now, I teach my clients how to do this too.
I even went on to hire a mindset coach in 2021, someone who has helped me more than I could ever possibly describe in words. Her mindset work took the work I was already doing each day to a new level.

The mindset coaching I've invested in and done has genuinely changed my life and changed who I am as a person. When I lean into these mindset practices, dig deep, and peel back those layers I've been hiding under my whole life, I feel like I am slowly becoming more myself with each passing day. I'm able to finally be honest with myself and recognize and honor my emotions head-on, versus stuffing them deep down. The funny thing is, when you stuff them deep down, they always seem to resurface in different ways, don't they?

This might be a little "woo-woo" for some of you, but I don't believe that anything I've accomplished or done in my life has happened by accident. I truly believe I have manifested everything that has happened over the last few years. It hasn't been luck. It hasn't been by chance. It's been because I've done the work to ask myself the hard questions, ask myself what I truly desire out of my life, ask for help, and take the action steps to get me closer to my goals. I've learned to think differently, and I've learned how to cope with my emotions and self-doubts. I'm not perfect, and I still have many layers to peel back, but I've finally gotten to know myself, and I've been pleasantly surprised to learn I like the person I am becoming.

I've never been a religious person, but this mindset journey has helped me realize that I am a spiritual person. It's let me learn to believe in myself in ways I never thought possible. It's allowed me to believe in the higher power of the universe and to know that what I desire truly is possible for me.

And it's possible for you too. So if you are consumed with worry, doubt, fear, and overwhelm—so was I. But you truly have the power to accomplish whatever your heart desires. But the first step is to start to believe that all of what you desire and more is possible for you too. I say this all the time: "Whether you believe you can or you can't, you're right." If you are constantly telling yourself that you are a failure and you will never hit your goals, then yes, that's exactly what's going to happen. But if you tell yourself that you can do hard things and that you will succeed, it's more than likely the actions you need to take to get you there will follow suit.

And if you're not buying into all that witchy, hocus-pocus BS, that's fine (I'll save the pixie dust for another time). Instead, I'd like to share with you the actual science behind why mindset work is so impactful and effective when it comes to long-term success and outcomes on this journey.

The Science Behind Mindset Work

You didn't really think I'd leave you high and dry without some facts to back all of this up, did you? Below are some mindset techniques that I have used personally and encouraged my clients and members to dive into to peel back those layers and truly recognize and acknowledge how they are feeling.

Mindfulness

Mindfulness is awareness. Mindfulness is the act of bringing attention and focus to our thoughts, behavior, and surroundings. Mindfulness is an effort to suspend judgments about the past and future and approach our thoughts and feelings from a place of curiosity. It can be practiced anytime, anywhere, and isn't limited to meditation or journaling.

People have been practicing mindfulness for thousands of years. The concept of mindfulness originated from Eastern religious and secular traditions—from Hinduism and Buddhism to yoga and, more recently, nonreligious meditation.[98] Practicing mindfulness can impact the body's cortisol, serotonin, melatonin, and epinephrine levels, which impact sleep, weight loss, digestion, stress, cognitive ability, attention, and a host of other physical and mental health symptoms.[99]

Anyone who has had weight loss surgery will tell you, it's a mind game! We can be our worst enemies and stand in the way of our progress. Addressing our mindset is key to being successful long term. We cannot be mindful of our eating and our habits when we are not caring for our minds first.

---

[98] JoaquÍn Selva, "The History and Origins of Mindfulness," Positivepsyhcology.com blog, published March 13, 2007, https://positivepsychology.com/history-of-mindfulness/.

[99] William C. Daube and Charles E. Jakobsche, "Biochemical Effects of Meditation: A Literature Review," *Scholarly Undergraduate Research Journal at Clark* 1, 10 (October 2015), https://commons.clarku.edu/surj/vol1/iss1/10/.

Journaling

Journaling has been scientifically connected to improvement in chronic mental health conditions. In a study where participants journaled for 10–15 minutes a day, 3–5 days a week, participants had fewer physical health symptoms, faster wound healing, increased health, better interpersonal relationships, higher quality of life, etc., in as little as one month.[100]

Here are a few more things journaling can do for you:

- Allow you to hone a growth mindset;
- Allow you to disclose and process feelings and emotions rather than stuff them down;
- Diminish pain or shame about feelings or events in your life and allow you to process them in a positive way;
- Bring awareness to your body, processes, and habits;
- Recognize trends or patterns in your thought processes;
- Recognize personal growth and non-scale victories;
- Address limiting beliefs

In a 2006 study, 100 adults journaled for 15 minutes twice weekly and saw a marked improvement in symptoms like anxiety and depression after only one month compared to the control group. When surveyed, 61% stated openly that they weren't comfortable with or "didn't like" journaling, and only 80% had journaled before.[101]

You don't have to like it, be comfortable with it, or even believe in it for journaling to work. And if journaling just really isn't something you can lean into, you aren't alone. There are other ways to practice mindfulness outside of just journaling. A few examples include

[100] Daube and Jackobshe, "Biochemical Effects."

[101] Kira M. Newman, "How Journaling Can Help You in Hard Times," *Greater Good Magazine*, published August 18, 2020, https://greatergood.berkeley.edu/article/item/how_journaling_can_help_you_in_hard_times.

- Saying your gratitudes out loud
- Writing them on a dry erase board or sticky note
- Exploring these concepts in meditation
- Reflecting while you lie in bed
- Using a voice note app or sticky note app on your phone
- Typing into a word processing document on your computer
- And so much more.

Yes, there are scientific benefits to journaling with a pen and paper. But don't get caught up in all-or-nothing thinking, especially when you are just getting started.

<u>Fixed vs. Growth Mindset</u>

In her book *Mindset*, Carol Dweck proposes that in a fixed mindset, we believe our basic qualities (intelligence, talent, athletic abilities, etc.) are fixed traits. In a growth mindset, we believe that our most basic abilities can be developed with time and effort.[102]

A fixed mindset could say, "I mindlessly ate a bag of chips again! I am never going to get this right. I am a failure."

A growth mindset could say, "I don't like that I ate that bag of chips mindlessly. I will think about why I did that so I can address some of the underlying things that are happening. Next time I want chips, I will put them on a plate with sliced cheese or some deli meat. I am not a failure. I am learning."

In a fixed mindset, everything is about the outcome. If you fail—or you're not the best—it's all been wasted. A growth mindset allows us to value ourselves and our journey, regardless of where we are on that journey. This can unlock incremental improvements, despite challenges and setbacks. It can also help

[102] Carol S. Dweck, Mindset: The New Psychology of Success (Ballantine Books, New York, 2016).

us be resilient when the comparison monster rears its ugly head. Working on practicing a growth mindset can be extremely empowering on a bariatric journey.

Gratitudes

Gratitude is "the quality of being thankful, a readiness to show appreciation for and return kindness."[103] How does practicing gratitude help us be more mindful? Gratitudes express appreciation for what we already have in our lives. They are an acknowledgment of value independent of monetary worth. Studies have shown that practicing gratitude makes us more likely to experience gratitude in the future. Areas in the prefrontal cortex of our brain gain heightened sensitivity to future experiences of gratitude the more it is practiced.[104]

Gratitude can improve feelings of inherent worth, positivity, and resilience. People who are grateful "feel less pain, less stress, suffer insomnia less, have stronger immune systems, experience healthier relationships, and do better academically and professionally." Gratitudes are a gateway to mindfulness techniques and can help us get in the right mindset for some of the more specific work we do in journaling.[105]

Limiting Beliefs & Affirmations

The things we believe are the lens through which we view the world. They can "influence perceptions, define what is good, bad, true, real, and possible, skew perspective in a positive or negative way, direct or limit the actions we take, shape character, affect relationships, determine health, and raise or lower happiness."[106]

---

[103] "Gratitude," *Oxford English Dictionary* online, accessed July 17, 2023, https://www.oed.com/view/Entry/80957?redirectedFrom=gratitude#eid.

[104] "Gratitude," "Thankfulness" section of PsychologyToday,com, accessed July 15, 2023, https://www.psychologytoday.com/us/basics/gratitude.

[105] Psychology Today, "Gratitude."

[106] Steve Sisgold, "Limited Beliefs: The Buzz Killer," "Dreaming" section of PsychologyToday.com, pub-

Limiting beliefs are things we believe about ourselves that limit our ability to reach our goals. While limiting beliefs may be informed by our life experiences, they are often not wholly grounded in reality and reflect fear, resignation, low self-esteem, and a lack of self-worth. Affirmations can be a powerful tool in overcoming limiting beliefs.

Participating in "positive self-talk *is* more than a confidence booster. From a neuroscience perspective, it might be more like internal remodeling."[107] So think about something you want to do in life. As you imagine the steps you need to take to get there, does your internal self-talk chime in with all the reasons why you can't? Now, let's talk back to that negative self-talk. Talk back to those limiting beliefs with affirmations.

For example, I struggle with making space for my personal goals, the goals that don't impact anyone but me, on my daily to-do list. So one of the affirmations I write when I journal is, "My goals have value and deserve to be a priority in my life." I think this comes from the limiting belief that if I am taking care of myself and prioritizing myself, then I am somehow being selfish or not doing enough for others. Logically, I know that that's not true at all! If anything, in order for me to be able to show up for the people in my life who I love and care about, I need to make sure I am filling my own cup first. This way, I am able to be the best version of me both for myself and for them.

We can logically know something, but subconsciously, it's hard to believe, which is why it's so important to do the work to start to reframe and rework that mindset.

Some Practical Ways to Start Working on Your Mindset

---

lished June 4, 2013, https://www.psychologytoday.com/us/blog/life-in-body/201306/limited-beliefs.

[107] Laura Starecheski, "Why Saying Is Believing—The Science of Self-Talk," "The Changing Lives of Women" section on NPR website, published October 7, 2014, https://www.npr.org/sections/health-shots/2014/10/07/353292408/why-saying-is-believing-the-science-of-self-talk.

Rewiring the Brain

The thing is, our brains are SO accustomed to thinking negative thoughts. What happens is, in plain terms, the neurotransmitters in your brain fire off and are used to following the same pathways (i.e., the same thought processes) they always have. In order to truly change your mindset, and therefore change your habits, thinking patterns, and behaviors as part of this journey, you absolutely have to start training your brain to think differently. And ultimately, that looks like training yourself to lift yourself up and be your biggest cheerleader, not your biggest critic.

When we think of self-care, a lot of us envision spa days or pedicures. But *true* self-care means taking care of your inner being, day in and day out. Mindset work is self-care in its purest form.

The Mindset Practice I Teach My Clients

If you want to get working on mindset work, here is the five-minute journal routine I have all my clients and members start with. This is a practice that my own coach, Jaime Mass, taught me when I started working with her. Most of my clients roll their eyes at me when I tell them their first goal is to journal before we even dive into their nutrition goals. But usually, by the end of our time together, they come back and thank me for "making them" journal (spoiler alert: I don't make anyone do anything! They chose to do that all on their own, and you can too!)

Not only is no one going to stick to a nutrition routine if they aren't simultaneously working on their mindset behind the habits, but setting mindset-driven goals is such a beautiful way to start building a consistent routine and getting yourself accustomed to sticking to a goal. If you can't commit to this 5–10 minute journal routine each day, how the heck are you supposed to commit to all the other time-consuming goals you will need to achieve on this journey? This routine helps get you geared for bigger goals along the way.

5–10 MINUTE JOURNALING ROUTINE:

Step 1: Gratitudes

The first thing I have people do is practice gratitude. I usually suggest they pick 2–3 micro and 2–3 macro gratitudes.

Micro Gratitudes: something you are grateful for that occurred just within the last 24 hours.

These gratitudes are super important, because it's really easy to disregard the "little" things in life and take them for granted. By reflecting back on the last 24 hours only, you are forced to be more present in your day-to-day life and appreciate the "small" things on this journey. If you know each day you are going to sit down and reflect on the previous 24 hours, it's going to force you to take better note of the things you're grateful for in the moment. Some of the things I find myself writing down look like this: snuggling with my dog in the morning, going to my early morning gym session, or watching TV before bed with my husband. Stopping to recognize what a privilege it is in my life to do those things allows me to appreciate the day-to-day routine a bit more.

Macro Gratitudes: something you are grateful for in your life as whole.

These are the gratitudes that are the more typical or bigger ones in life we think of. Some examples I often find myself being grateful for include my home, my health, my bariatric journey, my family, etc. Focusing on the macro gratitudes allows us to "zoom out," look at our life as a whole, remind ourselves of why we are working so hard toward our goals each day, and give ourselves a bigger purpose.

Step 2: Affirmations

Affirmations are probably my favorite part of my 5–10 minute journaling rou-ine. This is the part that often gives people that "impostor syndrome" and makes them feel like they are "lying" to themselves as they write. That's okay. This is because you are just beginning to reroute those neurotransmitters and create new thoughts in your brain. Affirmations can be in the form of "I am" or "I will" statements. They can also look like manifestations or mantras. Below are some of examples of affirmations I gravitate towards often:

- I am enough.
- I am getting better and better every day.
- I am strong and resilient.
- I wake up motivated each day.
- It is safe for me to be seen and heard.
- My goals are important and deserve time and attention.
- I am worthy and deserving of all the success I am experiencing.
- What I desire is already on its way to me.
- I am allowed to define my own success.
- I am good for other people.
- I am a good friend, and people can't wait to spend time with me.
- I deserve the same love I give to others.
- My goals are important.
- What is meant for me will not pass me.
- I do my best each day, and my best is enough.
- I believe in me.
- Incredible success is for people like me.
- I trust myself to show up and take action on the things I value most.
- I face my fears and build confidence by showing up anyway.
- This situation is difficult, but I have the skills and abilities to deal with it.
- I'm allowed to rest without guilt.
- I release the expectation I've put on myself to be "perfect."
- My obstacles motivate me to learn and grow.
- I love my body because it does many great things for me.
- I refuse to be undervalued by people around me.

- I trust my ability to navigate whatever life throws at me.

You can honestly turn anything you want to believe to be true into an affirmation. I suggest picking two or three that resonate with you and writing them down each day, until they no longer feel like "lies" you are telling yourself. What's really cool is, over time, you might find yourself naturally just thinking throughout the day "I am enough" or "I am capable of this." Once this starts to happen, it's alarming. It's like, "Oh my God, who just said that?" It's a really wild experience to go from not believing a statement you write down to having it just be a natural thought process. In addition to writing your affirmations, saying them out loud or recording yourself saying them and playing it back can be really effective too, since our brains recognize our own voices more than anyone else's. Pretty cool, huh?

Step 3: Limiting Beliefs

Limiting beliefs can sometimes be tricky. I've even had clients tell me reflecting on them sometimes brings up negative emotions. If leaning into or working through limiting beliefs feels like too much for you, that's okay; you can skip over them or work through them with a therapist or counselor.

The way I usually practice limiting beliefs is by first making a "T" chart. On the left side, I write out the "false" belief or narrative I keep telling myself. On the right side, I think of all the ways that it's actually not true or factual, as well as affirmations that can help me believe something different.

An example of this is the limiting belief I used to tell myself about my ability to run. I really wanted to start running, but I struggled to identify as being a "runner" and felt like I was "too fat" to run. Now, that wasn't true, but I had some pretty deep wounds from being made fun of in school when we used to have to run the mile in gym class, which led me to believe that I couldn't run, because I was "too fat." That was a very real experience for me at the time, which is why it was ingrained in my brain to think that thought. But that didn't mean it was still true all these years later.

Here is how I started to get out of that limiting belief:

Limiting Belief	Facts to Dispute It
1. I'm too fat to run.	1. I've lost 100+ lbs, and I'm no longer struggling with my weight. 2. Just because I couldn't physically run before doesn't mean I can't now. 3. I don't have to be fast to be a runner. 4. I have two legs that work well, and I am able to start running whenever I choose.

Step 4: Journal Prompts & Free Writing

Lastly, I like to encourage people to just free write and see what comes up. Simply ask yourself how you are feeling in that moment and see what comes up when you are honest with yourself.

If figuring out where to start is hard, here are some journal prompts I encourage people to lean into when they are getting started.

Pro tip: Go back and keep revisiting the same journal prompt over and over again as time goes on; usually, when it comes to peeling back these "layers," we need to ask ourselves these questions more than once!
(These sample journal prompts are meant to build on top of one another)

- What is your "why?" What is your reason for having surgery and venturing onto this journey?
- Who do you look up to most in your life? What qualities do they have

that are admirable? Do you have any of those qualities too?

- When you picture yourself at your goal weight, what does your life look like? Close your eyes and imagine you have accomplished EVERY goal on your bucket list.
- What are those goals? (Get specific!)
- How do you feel hitting those goals?
- What makes you most proud?
- How can you start doing those things and embodying those feelings now, despite the number on the scale?
- Which qualities does your future self have that have helped you get to your ultimate goals?
- Which traits do you need to let go of in order to get here?
- Which action steps are you taking every day in order to get to this dreamy place where all your goals and needs are met?
- What can you do today to take one small action or one step toward being that person who has hit all their goals?

The Truth about Happiness That No One Tells You on This Journey

I don't know who needs to hear this—well, that's a lie; I do know, as it's each and every one of you—so here it is: *weight loss does not bring happiness.* I want you to write that down somewhere and look at it each and every day.

The hard truth is, if you are waiting until the day when you hit a certain number on the scale in order to allow yourself to be happy, I worry you will be waiting forever.

It's a really sad and empty promise we tell ourselves:

"Oh, if I just hit this number on the scale, then I'll be happy."

"Once I lose just 10 more pounds, then I'll be happy."

"If I could fit into these jeans, then I would be so happy."

"Once I get a tummy tuck and all the loose skin removed, then I'll finally be happy."

I'm really sorry to burst your bubble, but no, no you won't. There is certainly a level of satisfaction that comes with hitting a goal, sure, and I truly am happier now in a smaller and healthier body, but in those first few years post-op, when I was at my then lowest weight and maintaining, it still never felt like "enough." I actually remember feeling really lost for a while. I felt like I didn't know who I was anymore.

I felt like my mission to lose weight had become my entire identity. From the time I was eight years old, I felt like my weight was always on the forefront of my mind, and since childhood, I'd been working towards losing weight.

One day, I was sitting in my therapist's office, telling her how I "just wanted to lose ten more pounds." I really didn't need to lose any more weight at the time, but in my head, I most definitely did.

I remember her saying, "Jamie, what if you are no longer the girl who has to lose weight? If you didn't have to lose weight anymore, who would you be?"

It was at that moment I burst into tears. I genuinely did not know. And it scared the hell out of me that I didn't know who I was without my identity as the "girl who needs to lose weight."

It might sound ridiculous, but for so many people, their identities get wrapped up in their weight and into their weight loss journeys. It's almost like your weight loss surgery starts to become a part of your personality sometimes. But bariatric surgery is something you *do*; it's not who you are.
I wish I'd had someone to tell me that losing weight wouldn't just magically solve all my problems or that it wouldn't be the thing that would transform me into the "me" I always wanted to be. Perhaps physically, yes; but mentally and

emotionally, I was exactly the same as I had always been, just more confused by what I saw on the outside.

So this is me giving you permission and encouraging you to work on your happiness and your mindset *now*. Please don't wait until you hit a number on the scale to allow yourself to be happy or to find joy in your life. You have to believe you are enough now, regardless of what that number on the scale or the tag on your jeans says.

Bite-Sized Recap

- Having bariatric surgery will likely bring up a lot of feelings.
- When you are struggling with feelings and emotions, *you cannot solve an emotional problem with a nutritional solution.*
- Mindset is a huge component to bariatric surgery and should not be overlooked. Weight loss surgery changes your anatomy and physiology, not your mindset. That part is on you.
- Mindset practices such as journaling, practicing affirmations & gratitudes, and writing out limiting beliefs can help you reroute the neurotransmitters in your brain to support you in making the necessary mindset changes and shifts to start to think differently after surgery.
- You don't need to wait until you lose weight to be happy. In fact, you should be working on creating happiness and joy in your life right now, as you lean into the process and change.
- You have to believe you are enough. And in case no one has told you this before I want you to know: you are enough.

For more journal prompts and resources related to this chapter be sure to head to www.thesleeveddietitian.com/easy.

Chapter 13
The Hard Stuff:
Mental Health & Addiction

men·tal health

/men(t)l/ /helTH/

noun

1. a person's condition with regard to their psychological and emotional well-being

"All this pressure seems to be affecting her mental health."

Trigger Warning: This chapter discusses mental health struggles in detail, including but not limited to: eating disorders and behaviors, depression, and anxiety. Please feel free to skip over this chapter if needed.

Mindset vs. Mental Health

I'd be doing you all a disservice if I let you believe that mindset work alone will just magically solve your problems. Overcoming obesity is a puzzle. Mindset work is just one piece of that puzzle. While mindset work can support you on your mental health journey, it can't replace actual mental health therapy, treatment, and support. So please don't think for one second that journaling or manifesting your affirmations is going to replace anxiety medications, anti-depressants, trauma therapy, or eating disorder treatment.

So many people struggle with mental health both before and after weight loss surgery, and I don't think it's talked about enough, nor do I think there is enough support given or awareness raised to bariatric patients about this. I think, due to weight stigma and bias, many people with obesity suffer from various mental health issues prior to surgery; but these issues fly under the radar, because people with obesity often don't receive the same level of treatment, empathy, and care as people in thinner bodies.

While most bariatric patients are required to undergo a psych evaluation prior to surgery approval in the US, as most bariatric patients will tell you, it's a very surface-level questionnaire. And to be honest, my psych evaluation was a joke. As someone who was a lifelong master at hiding how she felt and what she struggled with, I knew exactly what the psychologist was looking for me to say and not say. I wouldn't say I lied on my psych evaluation, but I certainly wasn't nearly as forthcoming with my struggles as I could have been. And perhaps that's on me. But I still think when going through a change as big as bariatric surgery, you should be required to attend more than just one, 20-minute pre-op evaluation.

And to make it worse, most bariatric patients aren't given adequate resources for finding a therapist who is well versed in surgery (and supportive of it). One of the most common questions I get is "Jamie, I have been looking for a therapist, but I don't know how to find one that is familiar with WLS." And to be honest? A lot of the time, I'm not even quite sure where to direct them either.

My Story

Over the years of sharing my WLS journey on social media, I've gotten pretty comfortable with being vulnerable with my struggles.

It's interesting though that, with as much as I've openly shared, the one thing I still find really hard to share and talk about is my eating disorder. It's something I don't talk about often and skim over whenever I do mention it or it comes up. To be honest, even typing out the words "my eating disorder" brings on a wave of impostor syndrome and old emotions. It's one thing for me to acknowledge I've struggled with disordered eating in the past, but to actually *accept* that I have struggled with—and will always have to work to overcome—a diagnosed eating disorder is still hard. I've been in a really good place for many years now, but still, admitting my past struggles makes me worry people will think I'm somehow a bad dietitian. (There are those limiting beliefs again!)

The thing about eating disorders is they never seem "bad enough" to warrant help. That's the disorder talking. And logically, I know what I went through was bad, but because I suffered through it while still at one of my heaviest weights, it never seemed bad enough. When you are thin and you develop an eating disorder, you are sent to the hospital. When you are obese and develop an eating disorder, people only see the weight loss and tell you to keep going and not give up. So that's what I did.

When people think about disordered eating in overweight people, they usually think of **BED (binge eating disorder)**. I'm not invalidating the severity of BED in any way, and I absolutely have struggled with binge eating throughout my entire life, especially as a kid and a teen. But I think it's important for people to know that eating disorders do not discriminate or come in a size.

In college, prior to studying nutrition, I lost 70 pounds for the first time "on my own." The first 50 pounds or so were lost in a pretty healthy way, I would say. I was being mindful of portions, and I wasn't cutting out food groups, just paying attention to how much I was eating. I was working out, drinking more water, and being consistent.

However, as that year came to an end, I had gained back about 7 pounds over the holidays. Looking back now, I know that really wasn't much or something to get too overwhelmed with. But at the time, it was absolutely horrifying and devastating to me. I REFUSED to let my hard work go to waste. The thought of going back to being as heavy as I was the year before scared the hell out of me.

But rather than just getting back on track with my routine, I decided to "go harder" than ever. What started off as healthy quickly turned into severe undereating. Eating less and less was becoming an obsession, as was working out.

I was going to school and working nights waiting tables at the time. In between classes, or before my evening and weekend shifts (which were spent on my feet for long hours, I might add), I was spending every moment I could at the gym, rarely taking a day off. And I was continually eating less and less. A typical day of eating for me looked like this: coffee in the morning, half an apple after the school day before my shift, maybe the other half of the apple when I got home or a few bites of a plain avocado. I remember eating the apple and feeling disgusted with myself for how "heavy" it felt in my stomach after running all day on empty.

The weird thing about eating disorders is they tend to shift and change shape in how they present themselves over time. When I was young I struggled with addictive food behaviors and binge eating. But at this time in my life, for the first time, having nothing was addictive. The less I ate, the more addictive the feeling felt. I can still remember the feeling of having nothing in my system for days and the power I felt I had within that feeling.

But of course, this wasn't sustainable or healthy in any way, and I slowly started to crumble. I didn't even realize what was happening at the time. All I knew was I no longer felt like myself. I felt like a shell of who I used to be, completely empty and removed from everything that made me feel like me. Looking back now, I realize it was a major depressive episode.

Not only was I not eating, but I wasn't sleeping. It was the strangest thing. I think when you deprive your body of food for months at a time, the way I did, all your bodily functions get confused. I couldn't sleep, and I think the insomnia coupled with the lack of food and energy is what caused the severity of the depression.

I also just felt angry all the time. I was constantly snapping at people around me. I would get so overwhelmed, especially around food, that I wouldn't know how to handle it, and I would snap. One time specifically, my mom took my sister and I out to lunch for a mother-daughter day. I ordered a dry salmon salad with no dressing. I intended to pick around the lettuce. When the waitress brought my salad, it was drenched in dressing. I don't know how to describe it, but seeing the dressing made me want to crawl out of my skin. I couldn't handle the thought of eating it. Instead of sending it back, I just didn't eat any of it. My mom was concerned and basically begged me to just eat it, but I couldn't. I ended up yelling at her. And I felt so bad. My mom was trying to do something nice and take us to lunch, and I couldn't even eat a bite of my salad. This was just one of many situations like this.

Luckily though, I was living at home, and my mom started to catch on to the fact that I wasn't acting like myself. She could see I was depressed and just not me. While I never went to any sort of outpatient (or inpatient) eating disorder treatment, I did start going to therapy at my mom's encouragement. But it still just never felt "bad" enough. Or rather, it didn't feel like my struggles were valid.

I remember telling my current therapist this a handful of years later. By the time I had transitioned to my current therapist, I was about a year post-op (and doing immensely better, as I had spent about four years in therapy prior to my VSG too).

I remember telling my therapist, "Well, yeah, I think I struggled with disordered eating a bit, but it's not like I actually had an eating disorder."

My therapist looked at me long and hard. She set her notebook down to the side and leaned in and said, "I'm concerned about the fact that you don't think you've suffered from an eating disorder."

I explained to her that no one had formally diagnosed me, and I never went to "official" treatment, nor had I ever been underweight. So it just didn't seem like I fit the criteria. It must not have been *that bad.*

She said, "Jamie, you do realize your other therapist referred you to me because

I specialize in eating disorders, right?" I looked at her blankly. She continued, asking, "If you had the formal label and diagnosis of an eating disorder, would it validate it for you?"

I nodded as she told me that it was in my chart that my previous therapist had forwarded to her. I don't know why having that label was validating for me, but it was.

Which Came First, the Chicken or the Egg?

Over the last 10 years, I've spent a lot of time working on my mental health and working with therapists, both before and after surgery. It's interesting though, because even though I overcame so many of my struggles before surgery, new ones have come up since.

It makes me wonder, were these new struggles always there? Did going through this journey just make me recognize them as I worked on my relationship with myself and food? Or did this journey and the hardships that come along with it bring about new struggles? Which came first, the chicken or the egg?

Mental Health Struggles I Experienced before Surgery

In addition to seeking out therapy for disordered eating prior to weight loss surgery, I also worked with my therapist on managing my anxiety. It wasn't until I was in therapy for disordered eating that I even realized I had anxiety—which is actually wild to me, looking back, because I've always been a highly anxious person. I ended up being diagnosed with **anxiety**, **OCD (obsessive compulsive disorder)**, and seasonal depression.

Mental Health Struggles I Experienced after Surgery

I would say the biggest struggle I've faced post surgery is the struggle with body dysmorphia. **Body Dysmorphic Disorder (BDD)** requires a clinical diagnosis and is defined as a mental illness involving obsessive focus on a perceived flaw in appearance.[108] My struggles with body dysmorphia didn't truly start until after my first round of plastic surgery.

In March 2020, I had my first round of plastic surgery to start the process of removing the excess skin after losing weight. I had a full abdominoplasty (tummy tuck) with muscle repair and a breast augmentation (implants). I then went on to have two more rounds of plastic surgery. In October 2021, I had a conversion from an abdominoplasty to a fleur-de-lis abdominoplasty to remove additional skin that was not able to be removed with the first tummy tuck, as well as a back lift for excess back skin. Lastly, in March 2022, I had a brachioplasty (excess skin removal on my arms).

It's interesting to me that I didn't experience body dysmorphia prior to these surgeries as badly as I did after. I think it was a combination of my body changing so drastically overnight combined with unrealistic expectations.

After losing so much weight, and still not being my happiest, I was convinced that having skin removal would be the end-all-be-all to achieving the happiness I had been waiting for. There was that empty promise again—once I do THIS, THEN I'll finally be happy.

I had it in my head that the reason I wasn't happy, despite my 112+ pound weight loss, was because of the skin. I had convinced myself that once the skin was gone, I would finally be happy with my body. It never even occurred to me that it could make my body image issues worse.

I just didn't look the way I imagined I would in my head. I've tried to describe how you feel after plastic surgery, and the best comparison I can give is that you wake up feeling like Frankenstein. You are nipped and tucked and pieced

[108] "Body Dysmorphic Disorder," "Diseases & Conditions" section of Mayo Clinic website, last updated December 13, 2022, https://www.mayoclinic.org/diseases-conditions/body-dysmorphic-disorder/symptoms-causes/syc-20353938.

back together in ways you don't recognize. And then, to make matters worse, other parts of your body stick out differently than they did before. For example: once my stomach was flat, and I didn't have a large apron of skin hanging over my midsection, I was suddenly incredibly aware of how "big" my legs looked compared to my now smaller waist, causing me to hyperfocus and fixate on the size of my thighs.

I don't regret any of my plastic surgeries, and I'm very grateful I've been able to have the skin removal surgeries I've had. But I wish someone would have prepared me for how hard they were going to be mentally. You can't go into plastics expecting to wake up looking like Barbie. It's just not how it works.

Where I'm at Now in My Mental Health Journey

About a year and a half ago, during one of my therapy calls, my therapist stopped me and said, "Jamie, are you nervous right now?"

"No, why?" I replied.

"Because," She explained. "You can't stop fidgeting. You do this often, but I've always assumed it's because you are nervous."

"No, I'm not nervous, I didn't even realize I was fidgeting." I said, a bit puzzled.

We started talking about how some of the things presenting in me as anxiety and OCD might actually be ADHD. However, as it turns out, getting diagnosed properly as an adult woman is a bit challenging. A year and half later, after a handful of psychiatrist appointments and evaluations, I was finally diagnosed.

Technically, ADHD is not a mental health condition, but a neurobehavioral disorder. However, for me, the symptoms of ADHD have intensely impacted the mental health struggles I do have, which is why I chose to add it to this chapter. It all ties in.

The interesting part? It wasn't until finally going on anxiety medications that I was able to receive a proper diagnosis of ADHD. It was pretty wild actually. Once we removed the intensity of my anxiety, and I wasn't constantly feeling the tightness in my chest from overwhelm, the behaviors that indicated ADHD worsened.

My therapist explained that my anxiety had been a coping mechanism for all of these years—that my anxiety was a way for me to ensure I didn't forget to do the things I needed to do. This is why, when my constant and debilitating anxiety eased, I noticed an increase in other struggles, including being late (time blindness), constantly misplacing things like my phone and keys, executive dysfunction (wanting to get things done, but feeling unable to do them), impulsivity, losing my train of thought, and hyperfixating on certain tasks while losing the ability to manage other tasks. The list goes on.

I've also learned ADHD is a spectrum disorder. My psychiatrist believes I may have once been lower on the spectrum, but with a growing business and less coping skills at my disposal, I've likely been pushed farther along on the spectrum, making it hard to mask and control my symptoms and struggles.

Because most ADHD studies primarily focus on males, and because ADHD presents in females differently than males, ADHD in females is often misdiagnosed. Please note that this is in direct reference to medical research that uses language that centers the gender binary, and you may identify with none or both of the symptom sets listed.

Most females don't receive a diagnosis until later in life (usually not until their 30s and 40s). And it's important to note that ADHD isn't something you develop over time; it's a lifelong struggle. So all of these women getting diagnosed later in life were just living with it unknowingly when they were younger.

Girls with ADHD tend to be less "hyperactive" than boys, and for girls, the behaviors and signs are less obvious. In girls, some of the symptoms might look like being a perfectionist, daydreaming quietly in class, feeling anxious or sad, silliness, acting shy or inattentive, trouble making friends, and picking at cuticles or skin.[109] Many girls with ADHD grow into women who are chronic overachievers with low self-esteem.

Want to know what else is interesting? A link has been uncovered between ADHD and obesity. People with ADHD tend to be low on dopamine, which is a chemical released in your brain that makes you "feel good." Because ADHD brains are low on dopamine, they are "chemically wired" to "seek more" according to John Ratey, M.D., professor of psychiatry at Harvard Medical School in Boston.

Ratey says, "Eating carbohydrates triggers a rush of dopamine in the brain" and that "It's the drive for the feeling of satiety."[110] This fact combined with impulse control issues, as well as low self-esteem, can be a recipe for disaster in women after weight loss surgery. It puts women with ADHD at a higher risk for BED.

According to a study at Duke University, it's estimated that nearly 30% of people who struggle with binge eating have a history of ADHD.[111] Binge eating disorder can leave people feeling out of control with food and experiencing immense shame and guilt, worsening their mental health struggles. Interestingly, people with ADHD are actually at higher risk for eating disorders in general, including anorexia, bulimia nervosa, and more.[112]

---

[109] Maureen Connolly, "ADHD in Girls: The Symptoms that Are Ignored in Females," "ADHD Symptoms & Tests" section of *ADDitude Magazine* website, published October 2, 2019, https://www.additudemag.com/adhd-in-girls-women/.

[110] Bob Seay and Nancy Ratey, "The ADHD-Dopamine Link: Whyy You Crave Sugar and Carbs," "ADHD Adults" section of *ADDitude Magazine* website, last updated January 21, 2023, https://www.additudemag.com/slideshows/adhd-obesity-link/.

[111] Sarah Haurin, "Understanding the Link Between ADHD and Binge Eating Could Point to New Treatments," *Duke Research Blog*, published March 18, 2018, https://researchblog.duke.edu/2018/03/13/binge-eating-disorder/.

[112] "Brain Reward Response Linked to Binge Eating and ADHD," ADHD Newsstand on Children and Adults with Attention-Deficit/Hyperactivity Disorder website, accessed July 15, 2023, https://chadd.

This all seriously makes me wonder—which came first? Did my struggles with early childhood obesity lead to my mental health struggles and my physical struggles with PCOS? Or did my struggles with ADHD and mental health lead to obesity and PCOS?

I'm not sure I will ever know. All I know, right now, is that none of this is a coincidence. And every struggle and hurdle I've had to work to overcome has led me to where I am now.

I'm still in therapy and on an anxiety medication, and I'm trialing ADHD medications as well. These tools, combined with the usage of Mounjaro, have made me feel that I can just breathe and think clearly for the first time in my life. Finally, for lack of a better word, I just feel "normal."

I've so badly needed all these pieces to fit together, and it all makes so much sense now. If my journey, which is just one unique example and experience, doesn't show you how complex obesity really is, then I don't know what does. There are just so many different layers: physical, metabolic, and hormonal issues, along with all the mental health pieces.

Our bodies are one singular unit. You can't focus on one "problem" and skip the rest. They are all entangled together. We can't possibly treat obesity with surgery alone. We must look at all of these other factors, pieces, and nuances too. You can't expect someone to be healthy physically if they aren't also healthy mentally.

Other Things to Consider in Regards to Mental Health after WLS

Antidepressant and Antianxiety Medications after Surgery

I have always been incredibly resistant to anxiety medications, mostly because I worried about the effects they might have on my weight. I was especially

org/adhd-news/adhd-news-adults/brain-reward-response-linked-to-binge-eating-and-adhd/.

resistant to them during the few years I spent struggling with regain. During that time, my anxiety seemed to skyrocket, and to be honest, I could have really used them. But I was already struggling with my weight, and I was not willing to go on an SSRI that might cause more weight gain.

I don't think enough attention is given to the fact that when people struggle with their weight and anxiety, it's a vicious circle. When you are anxious, it can exacerbate emotional eating and/or restricting and binging. It can also increase your stress and cortisol levels, making it harder to lose weight. Not being able to lose weight then furthers the anxiety. All the while, the idea of getting on an anxiety medication that may cause weight gain causes even further anxiety. See? One big, vicious cycle.

Personally? After being on an anxiety medication, I wish I could go back in time and kick past versions of myself for not getting on it sooner. I didn't know it was even possible to live the way I do now without constant, debilitating anxiety and overthinking. And getting the anxiety under control really helped me take the action steps I needed to in other areas (and of course, led to the ADHD diagnosis too). At the end of the day, what all of this has taught me is that I would rather be mentally healthy and be a few pounds heavier than struggle the way I once did.

Plus, one thing I came to learn is that you can advocate for yourself and talk with your doctors about which weight-neutral medications (meds that shouldn't affect your weight) may be an option. For so long I didn't tell my doctor that the reason I didn't want to go on an antidepressant was because I was worried about potential weight gain. But once I did, she heard me and validated my fears, and together, we explored options I was most comfortable with.

There are so many different mental health conditions (far too many for me to list here in this book) I know you and others may be struggling with. And taking medications for those diagnoses is SO important.

If you are on medication that affects your weight, make sure your PCP and your surgeon know. No one should be making you feel bad for not losing weight as quickly, or for regaining weight, because you are on medication.

And for whoever may need to hear this, you are not a failure because you need medication. Don't let anyone ever make you feel otherwise.

Addictions after Surgery

Addiction after surgery is perhaps one of the most important conversations to have in the bariatric space, yet it is one of the most overlooked.

There's still debate over whether or not one can truly have a "food addiction." Some researchers and practitioners argue that you "can't" be addicted to something that your body needs in order to survive. And while "food addiction" isn't included in the DSM (Diagnostic and Statistical Manual of Mental Disorders), there is overlap in the DSM-5 between substance use disorder and eating disorders.[113]

According to the American Society of Addiction Medicine, by definition, an addiction is "a treatable, chronic medical disease involving complex interactions among brain circuits, genetics, the environment, and an individual's life experiences. People with addiction use substances or engage in behaviors that become compulsive and often continue despite harmful consequences."[114] While addiction is most commonly associated with gambling, drugs, alcohol, and smoking, it's possible to be addicted to just about anything, including work, shopping, the internet/mobile devices, and more. So it's interesting to me that people still deny that you can be addicted to food. I see many professionals in the intuitive-eating space and HAES community, in particular,

[113] M. C. Rosa et al., "Overlap between Food Addiction and DSM-5 Eating Disorders in a Treatment-Seeking Example," *Drug and Alcohol Dependence* 166, 1 (November 2015: 192, https://nida.nih.gov/international/abstracts/overlap-between-food-addiction-dsm-5-eating-disorders-in-treatment-seeking-sample.

[114] "Definition of Addiction," Quality Care, American Society of Addiction Medicine, last updated September 15, 2019, https://www.asam.org/quality-care/definition-of-addiction.

taking the stance that one cannot be addicted to food; but I must say, as someone who has struggled with impulsive food behaviors and has worked with hundreds of people in the bariatric space, I can't help but disagree.

Either way, I think it's safe to say that many (certainly not all) bariatric patients have experienced addictive-like behaviors or personality traits, to some degree, and many people who undergo surgery label themselves as "food addicts."

So what happens when "food addicts" who don't receive treatment for their "addiction" are no longer able to eat large volumes of food?

Well, as you might suspect, the addictive behavior does not just go away or disappear. And unfortunately, post-op, many bariatric patients find themselves struggling with and facing **transfer addiction**.

A transfer addiction is when you can no longer engage in the addictive food behavior and, therefore, transfer said addiction to another behavior or substance. This is one of the reasons it's so important for bariatric patients to **avoid alcohol**, at least in the beginning phases of weight loss surgery. Personally, I don't suggest alcohol consumption, even moderately, until bariatric patients are 1) at least a 12+ months post-op and 2) have been working alongside a therapist who can closely monitor them if and when they add it back in.

Transfer addictions are very real, and I have seen them destroy and ruin lives. And they are not talked about enough, nor is enough support provided for them. Transfer addictions can be fatal—which is why if you are struggling with addiction-like personality traits, behaviors, and mental health issues, getting proper treatment is absolutely essential on your journey. I simply cannot stress that enough.

Emotional Eating after Surgery

While you may not be a "food addict," per se, you may still struggle with emotional eating. And just like with addictive behaviors, emotional eating behaviors won't magically disappear after surgery.

You may need to undergo intensive cognitive-behavior-change therapy and continue to work with a therapist long term to overcome or manage emotional eating behaviors. And while I'm not a therapist, and the tools and coping skills I can offer here (beyond the mindset skills I provided in the last chapter) are limited, I can confidently tell you this: don't overlook this one. I see too many bariatric patients ignoring emotional eating behaviors, only to find themselves still struggling after their surgeries, because the root of the issue was never addressed.

Eating Disorders after Weight Loss Surgery

Everyone's struggles are unique, and while my disordered eating improved through therapy, and I was able to keep those tendencies at bay after WLS, that isn't the case for everyone.

There are people who do, unfortunately, develop disordered eating habits after surgery, for a multitude of reasons. Similar to transfer addictions, disordered eating can occur post-op as a form of coping due to unresolved emotional struggles or traumas. For a lot of people, especially for those who may not have the proper pre- and post-op nutrition and emotional support, food and weight can become a hyperfixation after surgery.

It's important to recognize that eating disorders can develop as a result of weight loss surgery, and this is something that you absolutely deserve treatment for. If you notice you are struggling with obsessive food thoughts, behaviors, binging, purging, or restricting, it's important you reach out to your surgical team and/or your mental health practitioners for help.

Mental Health Matters

Mental health struggles, including eating disorders, are not contraindications to receiving obesity care via both medication and surgical bariatric interventions. However, they should be taken into consideration and monitored very closely by your medical and mental healthcare team.

Had I not had my weight loss surgery, many of my mental health struggles wouldn't have been found, addressed, or treated. I'm very grateful that my weight loss surgery brought them to light.

People can have mental health struggles and have surgery. People can also have surgery and then have mental health struggles. Obesity treatment isn't perfect, and making sure your mental health is at the forefront of your treatment plan is so important. If there is one thing you take away from this book, I hope it's the understanding that people who struggle with obesity are much more likely to struggle with mental health, making this journey all the more challenging. So be kind, always. You never know what someone is going through. And I hope each and every one of you, surgical patient or not, considers seeking out mental health therapy and treatment. It might just be the best thing you ever do.

Bite-Sized Recap

- While mindset work can support you on your mental health journey, it can't replace actual mental health therapy, treatment, and support.
- Mental health struggles are often experienced both before and after surgery. Sometimes new struggles pop up after surgery.
- Transfer addiction is a very real concern for people after weight loss surgery and should be taken very seriously.
- Emotional eating may continue to be a struggle for many after weight loss surgery and patients may need to undergo intensive cognitive-behavior-change therapy and continue to work with a therapist long term to overcome or manage emotional eating behaviors.
- Disordered eating behaviors can occur post-op as a form of coping due to unresolved emotional struggles or traumas. For a lot of people, especially for those who may not have the proper pre- and post-op nutrition and emotional support, food and weight can become a hyperfixation after surgery.
- Mental health struggles, including eating disorders, are not contraindications to receiving obesity care via both medication and surgical bariatric interventions. However, they should be taken into consideration and monitored very closely by your medical and mental healthcare team.

For journal prompts and resources related to this chapter, including how to find a therapist in your area, be sure to head to www.thesleeveddietitian.com/easy.

Chapter 14
Potential Barriers to Successful Surgery Outcomes: All the Nuances

dis·par·i·ty

noun

1. a difference in level or treatment, especially one that is seen as unfair

"economic disparities between different regions of the country"

Everyone Experiences Surgery Differently

No one surgery journey is the same. I don't think I truly realized this until I started working with WLS patients and taking on clients once I started my nutrition business.

Over the years, I've both created very meaningful friendships with various bariatric patients as well as taken on clients from various backgrounds. I've had friends and clients who were neurodivergent, Black, Hispanic, Asian, older, younger, people of all genders, and members of the LGBTQIA+ community. I've worked with people with disabilities, other chronic diseases, and ailments; people who have experienced immense losses and trauma; people who lived below the poverty line and people in the upper class; people with varying education levels; single moms; and parents of children with disabilities. I've also worked with people who had language barriers and who were hearing-impaired.

What I've come to realize is that not everyone is afforded the same opportunities to be successful and to receive the individualized support, care, education, and resources that they need in order to be successful.

Knowing obesity is a disease that is composed of environmental, genetic, and emotional factors, these are things that should be taken into consideration when someone is having surgery. So when the world says, "Just eat less and move more," or "Just work harder, stop with the excuses," all I hear is, "I'm so uneducated, ignorant, and oblivious to all the barriers and nuances that people struggle with that interfere with my one-size-fits-all suggestion."

None of these nuances are excuses. And they certainly aren't reasons one can't be successful with surgery. Of course, all these people can and are! These potential barriers are just extra things some people need to consider, address, or may need extra support with. I just don't think it would be fair to write a book about bariatrics told from the point of view of a White, heterosexual, cisgender female who lives in a two-income household without children, who is college educated, without acknowledging that my experiences are not universal to everyone. Now certainly, I've had my own barriers, as I've shared, when it comes to PCOS, mental health, and ADHD. So that's not to say that I, too, haven't had challenges; rather, the challenges I've faced might be vastly different from the challenges others have faced, and it's vital to include other perspectives too.

There are a lot of things people just don't think about when they consider going through weight loss surgery. This chapter is also going to talk about how one might experience WLS differently and face different struggles depending on different demographics, cultures, faiths, diagnoses, and general life circumstances. This chapter also addresses the way that these identities intersect with one another.

The amount of research, surveys, and studies done on the considerations below is alarmingly scarce. I had originally envisioned including many more facts and statistics in this chapter, but I had great difficulty finding studies and articles on these nuances. If that doesn't speak volumes to how underserved people with these struggles are, I'm not sure what does. So rather than giving you concrete numbers, instead, I am sharing with you my observations as well as allowing you to hear different patient stories and first hand experiences.

Nuances among Different Cultures, Races, Ethnicities, and Faiths

Language Barriers

If you are reading this, and English is your native language, I want you to imagine for a moment what it would be like to be presented with this book in Spanish. Or Italian. Or Chinese. Now I want you to imagine needing to read it and understand it. How likely would it be that you would be able to comprehend this entire book if it were in a foreign language? Not likely.

Just this past spring, in March of 2023, a study was conducted to evaluate the Spanish readability of ASMBS Centers of Excellence (COE) websites.[115] A Bariatric Surgery Center of Excellence means that "surgeons must be board-certified and demonstrate significant expertise in bariatric surgery. They must also stay abreast of the most current and appropriate treatments through ongoing continuing medical education."[116] The study acknowledges that healthcare disparities continue to be an ongoing struggle in the field of bariatrics.

The study found that 25% of COE websites were translatable to Spanish, concluding that Spanish readability of ASMBS COE websites is low.[117]

And what of other languages beyond Spanish? How is one supposed to make changes, follow guidelines, or even navigate the process of surgery if readable

[115] Theo Sher et al., "Evaluating the Spanish Readability of American Society for Metabolic and Bariatric Surgery (ASMBS) Centers of Excellence (COE) Websites," *Surgical Endoscopy* 37 (2023): 6395–6401, https://link.springer.com/article/10.1007/s00464-023-09978-9#citeas.
[116] Gary M. Pratt and Pam Greer-Ulrich, "Bariatric Surgery Centers of Excellence: Why They Are Important When Selecting Your Surgeon and Hospital," Obesity Action Coalition website, published Fall 2009, https://www.obesityaction.org/resources/bariatric-surgery-centers-of-excellence-why-they-are-important-when-selecting-your-surgeon-and-hospital/#:~:text=Keys%20to%20BSCOE%20Designation,through%20ongoing%20continuing%20medical%20education.
[117] Sher et al., "Evaluating the Spanish Readability."

and understandable resources aren't available?

Cultural Disparities & Considerations

Unfortunately, most healthcare providers don't have expansive cultural competency training. As a registered dietitian, between my four years of undergrad in nutrition and dietetics and my 1200+ hour clinical experience, combined with master's level classes in my dietetic internship, I received ONE lesson on cultural competency and awareness in nutrition coaching. Not one class, not one semester of material, ONE 45-minute PowerPoint presentation. And I know I'm not alone in this experience from an education perspective.

Too many bariatric patients are expected to abandon their cultural foods in pursuit of health. The unfortunate and discriminatory piece to this is, too many dietitians and healthcare professionals deem foods foreign to *them* as "unhealthy" simply because they don't know what these foods are.

Here's the reality: brown rice isn't superior to white rice. Bananas aren't superior to plantains. Quinoa isn't superior to rice and peas (black-eyed peas). And kale isn't superior to callaloo.

This all goes back to the fact that food isn't "good" or "bad," but simply different. So rather than telling a bariatric patient they "can't" eat the cultural and traditional foods they grew up on, how about we teach them how to eat these foods in ways that fit into their post-op bariatric routine?

It's incredibly unrealistic (and unnecessary) to demand a bariatric patient give up all of their cultural foods and food traditions. And as you've already learned here in this book, if it's unrealistic it's not going to stick or become a habit. The follow-through will be low. Bariatric patients who are told to forgo their cultural foods are put at a disadvantage compared to those who have the support with incorporating the foods that are culturally relevant and appropriate for them.

Laura, who is a previous client and current T.R.I.B.E.® member of mine says *"I have often felt like an outsider. I am half Chinese and half White. Having two cultural backgrounds I never felt "Chinese" enough or "White" enough. I am of a third culture that blends the two."* Laura identifies as a mixed-race woman who is Asian American and White, who is also neurodiverse, who had VSG in 2021.

She continued on to say:

> *Add the composition of my body—always being the biggest person in the room—I have struggled to see myself reflected in the media and communities I belong to. On top of that, people don't know what to make of me—guessing my background, asking questions or making assumptions that they wouldn't ask my white-presenting friends. I'm used to it but—depending on the day—am frustrated, sad, and outraged. But, more often than not, I feel alone. Even amongst my family (my siblings and first cousins are all mixed-race), we all have different relationships to our identities, informed by gender, sexual orientation, body composition, the neighborhoods we grew up in, ability, etc. We all "get it" but we all experience it differently too.*
>
> *When I made the choice to get bariatric surgery, I joined support groups hosted by my surgeon and didn't see anyone that looked like me or identified as Asian. It felt isolating, even though I didn't realize it at the time (to a certain degree, I'm used to it). I didn't feel seen or represented in discussions with my dietitian or in the materials given to us. Where were the bariatric versions of the food my grandparents gave me? How am I expected to give up noodles and rice? And no, brown rice is not the same. But my health was on the line, so I was willing to give up some of my culture, ties to my family, memories in consumable form. But I don't think the rotating parade of healthcare officials fully realized what they were asking.*

My memories of my grandpa who passed when I was 20, was of overflowing trays of chow mein. Standing next to him and his industrial sized wok as he made food for 50 people (and special treats just for me because I am his youngest granddaughter). Running into Chinatown shops to get ingredients. The day he taught me his secret batter recipe. There is legacy, tradition, and memories. And I know this is the case for many cultures, but in the materials I was given I saw bariatric versions of meatballs, tacos, Carne asada, and burgers. (All basic and stereotypical, and not without their limitations.) But what about char siu? Lemon chicken? Chow mein? Stir fry with black bean sauce? Instead I was told for the rest of my life I could eat an ounce of brown rice. But I should probably have cauliflower rice instead.

T.R.I.B.E. helped me feel less alone. The support from dietitians and other members was literally game-changing and made so much difference in my journey. Especially hearing from Jamie Mills and Melissa De Los Santos [Registered Dietitians in the T.R.I.B.E. program] that I can have rice and don't have to give up my culture. And I haven't. If anything, I eat more Asian food now than I did before. But I didn't feel truly seen until I befriended another mixed-race Asian American woman on Instagram and in the T.R.I.B.E. program. We chatted a bit and then found we have so much in common. We're close in age, close in weight loss, share similar points of view, love tattoos and travel. We joke that we're twins. And yes, we talk about being Asian American, about weight loss. But we also talk about our families and big life events. I don't have to tell her how it feels to be Asian American and a bariatric patient. She lives it too. Her experiences are hers and are different from mine, but the intersection of being a bariatric patient (and formerly larger bodied) and Asian American is something she understands and we share. Which makes this whole process a lot less lonely.

I wonder how different Laura's experience might have been, had the dietitian or surgeon from her surgery center supported her in adding these foods in usng a method like the bariatric meal plate. Or had she had the opportunity to meet her "bariatric twin" sooner on this journey. While I'm glad she made her way to the T.R.I.B.E.® and has since been able to add her cultural foods back in, she shouldn't have had to be made to feel like she had no other alternative than to simply give up all the foods she grew up on.

Racial Injustices and Disparities

According to the CDC, "Racism—both interpersonal and structural—negatively affects the mental and physical health of millions of people, preventing them from attaining their highest level of health, and consequently, affecting the health of our nation."[118] The CDC also states

> The data shows that racial and ethnic minority groups, throughout the United States, experience higher rates of illness and death across a wide range of health conditions, including diabetes, hypertension, obesity, asthma, and heart disease, when compared to their White counterparts. Additionally, the life expectancy of non-Hispanic/Black Americans is four years lower than that of White Americans.[119]

Seeing as all of these comorbidities coincide with obesity itself, it's not even a question that disparities within our healthcare system have made their way to those receiving bariatric care and treatment, or rather, prevent those from receiving adequate bariatric care and treatment.

A 2020 study found that "Black [bariatric patients] have higher odds of readmission and multiple grades of complications (including death) compared with White patients. Hispanic patients have higher odds of a Grade 3 complication [requiring surgical, endoscopic, or radiological intervention] compared with White patients."[120]

---

118 "Racism and Health," "Health Equity" section of CDC website, last updated November 24, 2021, https://www.cdc.gov/minorityhealth/racism-disparities/index.html.

119 CDC, "Racism and Health."

120 Leonard K. Welsh et al., "Racial Disparities in Bariatric Surgery Complications and Mortality Using

Another study performed in 2022 found that despite being eligible for bariatric surgery, based on both BMI and obesity-related comorbidities, African American men are significantly less likely to undergo bariatric surgery. And of the African American men who do receive surgery are found to be significantly younger than White men but also experience greater comorbidities compared to White men and all women.[121] They also found that compared to White men, African American men had a higher BMI, were more likely to have a history of hypertension, renal insufficiency, required dialysis, and were more likely to suffer from postoperative complications compared to White men.[122]

According to another study performed in 2022, "Recent studies have highlighted racial disparities in perioperative outcomes, including up to a two-fold higher mortality rate in non-Hispanic Black vs. non-Hispanic White patients. Causality for these disparate outcomes remains unclear and largely unexplored."[123] Their research found that one of the factors was an increased prevalence of postoperative venous thromboembolism, but more research is needed to further explore the reasons for this.

Another factor to consider is the racial bias that exists in the treatment and management of pain. It's pretty disgusting that people of color are less likely to receive adequate pain management, which can lead to poorer health outcomes.

In the 2021 study performed by the New England Journal of Medicine, researchers found that in "90% of the 310 health systems studied, the opioid dose prescribed to White patients was higher than the one prescribed to Black patients. On average, White patients received 36% more pain medication by

the MBSAQIP Data Registry," *Obesity Surgery* 30, no. 8 (2020): 3099–3110, https://www.ncbi.nlm.nih.gov/pmc/articles/PMC7223417/.

[121] A. B. Hoffman et al., "Disparity in Access to Bariatric Surgery among African-American Men," *Surgery Endoscopy* 34, no. 6 (June 2020): 2630–2637, https://pubmed.ncbi.nlm.nih.gov/31385077/.

[122] Hoffman et al., "Disparity in Access."

[123] Michael A. Edwards et al., "Racial Disparities in Reasons for Mortality following Bariatric Surgery," Journal of Racial and Ethnic Health Disparities 10 (February 2022): 526–535, https://link.springer.com/article/10.1007/s40615-022-01242-5.

dosage than Black patients, even though both groups received prescriptions at similar rates."[124] I don't know about you, but reading that statistic is completely jarring.

Alyssa Gomez, another client of mine, and a T.R.I.B.E.® member, speaks out about the impact of inequality in medical treatment and pain management. Alyssa identifies as a Mexican, heterosexual, cisgender female who is a nurse practitioner (NP).

Alyssa says:

> *I am a medical provider, a nurse practitioner who sees a vulnerable population of patients in chronic pain. I know what it sounds like when a provider cares and listens to their patients. I strive to be that for my patients. I never want them to feel how I feel, as if what I feel or say doesn't matter. I never want to mute my patients. I teach them to advocate for themselves.*
>
> *I will say that during my hospital stay after surgery, I was very vocal about my pain and needed my pain to be managed appropriately. At first they did not want to give me opioids, but I was in significant pain, and walking, Tylenol, and Gas-x were not touching it. I did bring up at that point that I was a NP in pain management and then finally my pain was addressed appropriately.*
>
> *There is a bias in life towards people of color, especially in healthcare. Being a female person of color, specifically a Mexican woman, I feel as though my voice has been lost or not heard through this surgical process. With my RNY surgery, I have never felt any restriction. I could eat a whole medium pizza if I wanted to, though I have been choosing not to.*

---

[124] Nancy E. Mordent et al., "Racial Inequality in Prescription Opioid Receipt—Role of Individual Health Systems," *New England Journal of Medicine* 385, no. 4 (July 2021), https://www.nejm.org/doi/full/10.1056/NEJMsa2034159.

I have tried countless times to meet with my bariatric surgeon to go over my questions and requests but still to this day have not been able to have any follow-up after my surgery with my surgeon. Every message from him is dismissive, not reassuring, and it feels as if he thinks I am making it up, that it's not possible for me to be able to eat that much so early on. He will send me a picture of the pouch he created on the day of surgery but not answer when I ask to be scoped for a current view of my pouch. My voice has been lost through this process, and it is at a point where I don't even bother anymore. Sometimes I wonder if I was a "White woman," would my surgeon hear me or take what I say under consideration?

I would have loved to be able to actually see my surgeon or a NP/PA in person since surgery. I have had many questions and concerns that still have not been addressed. If it wasn't for T.R.I.B.E. and the support I received, I would have been lost after surgery.

Alyssa shouldn't be taken any less seriously than anyone else when it comes to expressing her concerns or pain. And it's completely unacceptable that not only will her surgery center not allow her to come in for follow-ups, but that she needs to justify her needs by explaining she is a NP. She shouldn't only be taken seriously because of her credentials. She should be taken seriously, period.

There's a LOT of work to be done in order to make bariatric surgery more equitable and accessible for all as well as a LOT of work to be done to improve healthcare outcomes for people of color after surgery. Why are so few people talking about this and turning a blind eye?

Religion, Faith, and Traditions

Along with taking peoples cultural, ethnicity, and race into the conversation when it comes to nuances after surgery, one's religion, faith, and traditions are important to discuss as well.

Religion, which is a subset of one's culture, needs to be taken into consideration when having surgery. Everything mentioned above in regards to cultural food practices also applies to foods, meals, and traditions that take place amongst various religions.

Many faiths practice prolonged fasting, food-related rituals and traditions, and more, which can play a role in one's habits, care, and health outcomes after surgery.

According to the ASMBS the majority of published research on the effects of religious fasting covers the effects on adults who have not undergone weight loss surgery. Based on the review they conducted in April of 2022, the ASMBS suggests following these suggestion below prior to prolonged religious fasting:

- WLS patients follow-up with their surgeon and interdisciplinary team prior to fasting.
- WLS patients who also have diabetes are encouraged to consult with their clinicians to make appropriate medication adjustments.
- WLS patients who want to fast should be prescribed a proton pump inhibitor (medication to reduce acid secretion) to be taken daily for the duration of the fasting period. For example, patients fasting during Ramadan have been reported to complain of new-onset or exacerbated existing GI complaints, the most common complaints being dyspepsia (upper abdominal burning sensation) and heartburn (acid reflux).
- WLS patients should drink adequate liquids of >1.5 L/day (50oz) to maintain adequate hydration while fasting.
- While fasting, limit intake of sweets and foods high in saturated fat when breaking fast to avoid dumping syndrome and to avoid contributing to potential dehydration.
- Aim for nutritionally balanced meals pre or post fasting that include whole grains and lean proteins with a minimum of 60g protein/day.
- At the post-fasting meals, instead of having one large meal, aim for smaller more frequent meals during eating times in order to hit protein goals and avoid overfilling the pouch.
- Continue to take recommended dosages of vitamin and mineral sup-

plements as prescribed.[125]

Meeting nutritional needs after surgery can be quite difficult without the additional hurdles that come with prolonged fasting periods. It's incredibly important to follow up with your surgical team to come up with a safe plan if you are going to fast for religious purposes. As a side note, I do think it's important to mention that unless fasting is due to one's faith or cultural traditions, prolonged periods of fasting (such as Intermittent Fasting where one purposely restricts their eating during certain time periods daily) are not recommended for bariatric patients. Fasting also should not be used as a weight loss tactic after surgery.

Nuances between Varying Genders, Identities, and Those Within the LGBTQIA+ Community

I think one of the most interesting statistics when it comes to bariatric surgery is that only 20% of WLS patients are cisgender men.[126] I think this is especially interesting knowing that less than 1% of the entire population who qualifies for WLS takes advantage of it.[127]

When it comes to severe obesity, by clinical standards, cisgender men are less likely to suffer from it than cisgender women. About 1 in 11 adults (9.2%) have severe obesity. The percentage of cisgender men who are overweight (34.1%) is higher than the percentage of cisgender women who are overweight (27.5%), however, the percentage of cisgender women who have severe obesity (11.5%) is higher than the percentage of cisgender men who have severe obesity (6.9%).[128] But even still, for only 20% of all eligible cisgender men to be

125 Lillian Craggs-Dino et al., "American Society for Metabolic and Bariatric Surgery Review on Fasting for Religious Purposes After Surgery," *Surgery for Obesity and Related Diseases* 18 (2022): 861–871, https://asmbs.org/app/uploads/2022/06/PIIS1550728922001885-FASTING.pdf.

126 Sherif Aly et al., "Gender Disparities in Weight Loss Surgery," *Mini-Invasive Surgery* 4, no. 21 (2020), https://misjournal.net/article/view/3404#:~:text=Of%20the%20810%2C999%20patients%20who,loss%20surgery%20among%20eligible%20patients.

127 ASMBS, "Obesity in America."

128 "Overweight & Obesity Statistics," "Health Statistics" section of National Institute of Diabetes and Digestive and Kidney Diseases website, last updated September 2021, https://www.niddk.nih.

aking advantage of surgery, seems very low.

Ne still don't know exactly why this is. It's more than likely a multi-ude of factors. In general, it appears that cisgender men are less likely to each out for help or support until their comorbidities have progressed.

And I think that's very telling, right? We live in a society where cisgender men are still shamed for seeming "weak" or showing emotion or asking for help or support. And after surgery, there seems to be even less support available to cisgender men than cisgender women. The bariatric community, especially on social media, where many go for community and support, is largely made up of cisgender women, making most of the support option catered to other cisgender women.

And for full transparency, I personally feel caught between a rock and a hard place with this. As a dietitian who advocates for the community and works hard to provide adequate support, my programs are primarily focused on supporting women, those who identify as women, and gender-nonconforming people. And why is that? Because in the past, I had no cisgender men to offer my services and support *to*. So how do we offer more support for men if they aren't having surgery, but how do we help them take the steps to have surgery if they don't believe they are in need of or deserving of support?

There are also a lot of nuances and potential barriers to successful surgical journeys and outcomes amongst transgender bariatric patients. According to a 2019 review, "A Review of Psychosocial Risk Factors Among Transgender Patients Seeking Bariatric Surgery," despite ⅓ of transgender people suffering from obesity, "there is no research on transgender bariatric surgery candidates."[129] However, in the review article they bring up important nuances

gov/health-information/health-statistics/overweight-obesity#:~:text=More%20than%201%20in%20 3,who%20are%20overweight%20(27.5%25).

129 Lisa Hecht et al., "A Review of Psychosocial Risk Factors among Transgender Patients Seeking Bariatric Surgery," Obesity Surgery 29 (2019): 3365–3370, https://link.springer.com/article/10.1007/ s11695-019-04076-z.

and considerations for transgender bariatric patients including high rates of "mood pathology," substance use, abuse, and self-harm behaviors and potential psychosocial risk factors, including sex hormone management, which may impact surgical clearance, pre-surgical psychosocial assessment, and treatment recommendations.[130]

One of the things we talk a lot about in the bariatric community is the way dynamics shift and change after bariatric surgery and massive weight loss. These changes in relationship dynamics, and in some cases, the loss of a spouse or significant other who may not be supportive, etc., can really have an impact on overall outcomes or struggles on the bariatric journey. But how, if at all, does that change amongst the LGBTQIA+ community?

One of the nuances that has been presented to me many times during support groups is the struggles that arise within same-sex relationships. Society puts a lot of pressure on women's bodies, and an emphasis on changing bodies to be smaller. This can create rifts within same-sex relationships between women, especially if the bariatric patient's spouse struggles with weight too. Feelings of resentment may arise, and it might be different than the way resentment presents itself in other relationships.

Nuances among Different Diagnoses, Mental Health Conditions, and Abilities

While I won't dive too deep into mental health conditions here, as there is a whole chapter dedicated to the importance of mental health before and after surgery, it's important to realize, and for me to continue to emphasize here, that struggling with mental health can be a HUGE barrier to successful surgery outcomes.

Physical health conditions can also be huge barriers for bariatric patients. Many bariatric patients do have additional physical health conditions, espe-

130 Hecht et al., "Psychosocial Risk Factors."

cially taking into consideration many, if not most, WLS patients have or have had comorbidities leading them to surgery.

I've worked with dozens of bariatric patients who had dual diagnoses, including multiple sclerosis (MS), fibromyalgia, lupus, rheumatoid arthritis, Celiac disease, Graves disease, Hashimoto's, postural orthostatic tachycardia syndrome (POTs), just to name a few.

Each one of these physical health conditions presents its own daily challenges. On top of all the things bariatric patients need to do and manage, people with additional conditions and ailments have those health symptoms and treatments to manage in conjunction.

While doable, some of these diseases and disorders will make certain bariatric guidelines that much harder to abide by or be consistent with. Kind of hard to be consistent with working out each week or planning your meals when you have an autoimmune flare-up and can't get out of bed or leave the house.

Neurodivergent Folks & Disabilities

Neurodivergent WLS patients may also encounter unique challenges in their journeys. "Neurodivergent" is a term that describes people whose brain differences affect how their brain works.[131] People who are neurodivergent have various strengths and challenges that are different from people whose brains don't have those differences. Some of these differences may include medical disorders, learning disabilities, and other conditions.[132]

Some of the most common conditions people who are neurodivergent might have include autism spectrum disorder, attention deficit hyperactivity disor-

[131] "Neurodivergent," "Health Library: Symptoms" section of Cleveland Clinic website, last updated June 2, 2022, https://my.clevelandclinic.org/health/symptoms/23154-neurodivergent#:~:text=The%20term%20%E2%80%9Cneurodivergent%E2%80%9D%20describes%20people,learning%20disabilities%20and%20other%20conditions.

[132] Cleveland Clinic, "Neurodivergent."

der (ADHD), dyscalculia (difficulty with math), dysgraphia (difficulty with writing), or dyslexia (difficulty with reading) to name a few.[133]

All of these come with their own sets of challenges and potential need for accommodations or additional support. I've had many clients with ADHD, and I've given you my own perspective having it myself. Some of the most common challenges I see amongst my bariatric patients with ADHD are struggles with impulse control when it comes to food choices and habits. Time blindness, another common symptom of ADHD, where one struggles to keep track of time or struggles to estimate how long it may take to accomplish a task, may translate to struggles with remembering to take their vitamins, hit their protein goals, or drink their water on time throughout the day.

Bariatric patients who are neurodivergent, often those who have autism spectrum disorder, are often faced with challenges when it comes to meeting their nutritional needs due to various food aversions, often related to hypersensitivity to textures. Many people with autism are highly selective eaters and are often limited to the foods they are able to tolerate and eat.

Again, none of these things are reasons not to have surgery, nor are they reasons why someone can't be successful. It just means those people might need additional support in various areas in order to find a routine that works for them and will allow them to meet their needs. It's challenging enough to advocate for yourself in a medical setting when you struggle with obesity without having the additional challenges of neurodiversity, and potential mental and or physical disabilities.

The Main Point

It would simply be impossible to cover every single nuance under the sun, but I hope this chapter helps you see things from some different perspectives. I hope this chapter has expanded your ability to empathize with others. So

[133] Cleveland Clinic, "Neurodivergent."

Instead of telling people to just eat less and move more or berating people for taking the "easy way out," can we all just acknowledge that obesity and weight loss surgery are really f*cking hard? And that, sometimes, it's even harder for other people who are already at a disadvantage? Or have less access to individualized support based on their unique needs? Or aren't treated with equity?

The same goes for judging one another within this community. You have no idea what it's like to walk in someone else's shoes. So if someone is struggling, not hitting their goals, etc., we need to look at them with empathy and understanding, not judgment or pity. Because you have no idea what it's like to walk this path in their shoes, even if you know what it's like to walk in yours.

Bite-Sized Recap

- Everyone experiences weight loss surgery differently.
- Not everyone is afforded the same opportunities to be successful and to receive the individualized support, care, education, and resources that they need in order to be successful.
- There are SO many nuanced situations and circumstances that different bariatric patients go through. None of these nuances are excuses. And they certainly aren't reasons one can't be successful with surgery. Of course, all these people can be and are! These potential barriers are just extra things some people need to consider, address, or may need extra support with.
- Nuanced situations that can have an impact on surgery outcomes include, but are not limited to, varying cultures, races, ethnicities, faiths, genders, identities, sexuality, and mental and physical abilities.
- If someone is struggling, not hitting their goals, etc., we need to look at them with empathy and understanding, not judgment or pity. Because you have no idea what it's like to walk this path in their shoes, even if you know what it's like to walk in yours.

For journal prompts and resources related to this chapter be sure to head to www.thesleeveddietitian.com/easy.

Chapter 15
Gaps in Our System & The Work Ahead of Us

gap

/gap/

noun

1. a break or space in an object or between two objects
“Taking a seat on the opposite end of the room, her doctor made no effort to reduce the gap between them.”

2. an unfilled space or interval; a break in continuity
“There are many gaps in our postoperative support process.”

Time to Bridge the Gap

I think one of the most beautiful parts about being both a registered dietitian and a bariatric patient is I truly get to see things from all angles. I get to experience surgery and post-op life first hand as a bariatric patient, and I also get to experience it as a healthcare professional and practitioner.

I think because of this unique perspective, I have the ability to understand where patients might feel misunderstood, under-supported, or even confused with the things that are being asked of them, while simultaneously understanding frustrations and limitations from the clinical perspective.

One of my greatest missions is to help bridge the gap between patient and practitioner. I feel it’s my job to advocate for both the patient and the surgery center. When clients come to me, it’s my job to not just validate their frustrations and support them, but to encourage them to stay in communication with their care team and to advocate for themselves during their pre- and post-op appointments. Ultimately, if we can get these two groups to speak each other's language, we can avoid a lot of miscommunications and misunderstandings and fill the gaps in the system so that more patients can have better outcomes.

What I Noticed Was Missing

As I went through my own bariatric journey, I think the number one thing I noticed was missing was support. As a bariatric patient, I felt like I needed more support than my center could provide. But as a dietetic intern, when I was interning at a bariatric center at a local hospital, I could completely understand where and why even the best-intentioned practitioners struggled with things slipping through the cracks.

In this chapter, I'm going to talk about where I see some major gaps in the bariatric process, both before and after surgery, and where I see room for improvement and growth. These are solely my opinions based on my experience, the numerous anecdotal experiences I have heard from many of the bariatric patients I have worked with and spoken to, and the conversations I've had with many of my bariatric colleagues. This chapter is not meant to attack anyone or accuse anyone of poor care, nor is it meant to generalize all bariatric centers, practitioners, or methods. Rather, this chapter is meant to help my fellow clinicians and healthcare professionals see where we could all work together to improve the quality of care we provide to our patients and clients and see how we can all work to make sure bariatric patients receive what they need to be successful.

Preoperative Gaps

I will say, I think there are far fewer gaps in the pre-op phase as opposed to the post-op phase. In my experience, I feel like there is a lot more "hand-holding" before surgery versus after. Normally, at most centers, there is a bariatric coordinator who is able to help ensure you get all your appointments and sessions scheduled to make sure things go smoothly, and so you are able to stay on track for getting your surgery within the three to six month pre-op period.

I think the biggest pre-operative gap I see is lack of education. Despite required pre-op classes and nutrition sessions with dietitians, there still is so much confusion when it comes to what the post-op diet should consist of. I mentioned this in Chapter 9 as well, but I really believe the lack of understanding of the educational materials is due to patients only being told what to do, rather than also why and how they should do the things being asked of them.

There is just SO much to grasp and understand when it comes to preparing for life after surgery; I just don't feel like three to six 30-minute nutrition sessions is enough to grasp it all. And that's being generous—I've spoken to numerous people who have shared with me that they only met with a dietitian one time before surgery, or that their center and/or insurance didn't require nutrition visits. This also occurs sometimes when people are self pay and the nutrition visits aren't a requirement by insurance. In that case, if the surgery center doesn't require it, and the patient doesn't want to pay for it, it's likely they won't receive much beyond a binder of materials to look over.

Another gap I see, and also experienced during this phase, was a lack of emotional support. This time period is very stressful and overwhelming. Unfortunately, most people don't receive much support in this arena, unless they have willingly sought out their own therapy.

Postoperative Gaps

I think the greatest area for improvement lies within post-op care. There are definitely some hurdles with this. Unlike in the pre-op phase, it's hard for bariatric centers to enforce post-op visits. Unless the patient is willing to come to post-op visits, there really is no means to enforce them.

However, what I hear most often from bariatric patients is that they wish they had more post-op visits and that the surgeons and dietitians at their center were more available to care for them.

Typically, most centers see people at one to two weeks post-op, three months post-op, six months post-op, nine months post-op, 12 months post-op, and then yearly thereafter or on an as-needed basis.

Unfortunately, though, I have heard horror stories from patients who have told me that they aren't able to see their surgeons or dietitians at all. And no, not because of insurance battles (although that can happen), but because their center outright refuses to see them. I know; I was shocked when I heard this too. But this isn't an isolated experience. I've had many people tell me that when they call their center, either no one answers the phone or gets back to them or their center refuses to see them, telling them, "You're not a patient anymore. You already had surgery" or "That's an issue for your PCP." (Spoiler alert! Most of the time, when bariatric patients request to see their bariatric team, it's for a bariatric-related concern!) The thing is, once you have bariatric surgery, you are a bariatric patient for life, and you absolutely should be able to make an appointment with your surgical team whenever you need to. And it's terrible that that's not always the case.

After having so many pre-op appointments and being in such close contact with your bariatric team for so long, it can feel really lonely once you no longer are seeing them or receiving their support or care. And if anything, we require just as much, if not more, support after surgery than we did before. Once you have surgery, there is no going back, and you immediately need to make all the changes you've been gearing up for. But oftentimes, you won't know what you are going to struggle with or be confused and overwhelmed by until you have had surgery and are going through the process.

A lot of people feel like they've been dropped like a hot potato after surgery. It's like they say, "Okay, great. We took your stomach. Now, here's your binder with all the information you need. Good luck to you. Go forth and be happy figuring it out on your own!" Obviously, that's not what's said, and that's usually not what your bariatric team intends for you to feel or experience, but I know it felt that way for me, and it's felt that way for the vast majority of patients.

Most bariatric centers do offer support groups, and many patients are required to attend. I've discussed with many fellow dietitians and surgeons how to optimize the support groups at their weight loss centers, because historically, most WLS centers tend to experience pretty low attendance for their support groups. As someone who has been IN those support groups, I can tell you why that is: they usually aren't true support groups. They're usually lectures.

In my membership program, we offer over 40 live Zoom support groups every single month, and usually, we have a full house with upwards of 50 participants for EACH of those 40 groups. So I can tell you, it's not that patients don't WANT the support. They do, and they are more than willing to show up to receive it. So if they aren't showing up, it's likely because they aren't receiving what they're needing.

To everyone reading this who plays a hand in running or planning support groups, I'm going to let you in on a little tip: no one wants to go to a support group where they feel like they are being lectured at. I'm a firm believer that support groups should not involve PowerPoint slides or education materials. If that's what you want to provide, then call it what it is: a webinar, a lecture, a presentation, etc. Obviously, proper education is important. I just mentioned there isn't enough of it, usually in the pre-op stages, but support and education are two different things. Someone can know what to do and struggle to do it. More education won't fix that, but support will.

Support groups are meant to be a place where meaningful discussions can take place. They aren't supposed to be a time to learn something new—or worse, learn something they've heard a million times over. When you're sitting there, struggling with all the emotional hurdles that come alone with weight loss surgery—struggling to believe in yourself and scared out of your mind you're going to "fail" again—and you show up to lecture about the importance of fiber or exercise, it honestly starts to give you flashbacks to Weight Watchers groups. It's not helpful. It's not enjoyable. And it really doesn't address the biggest concerns your patients have, which is how to address their fears and worries.

When you lead a support group, your role as the support-group leader is to manage and facilitate the conversation. That's it. You're not there to tell people what to do or give advice beyond maybe some general feedback. The purpose of support groups is to help people speak up, share their concerns, thank them for being open, validate their feelings, and encourage those around them to offer support or words of encouragement. THIS is how you provide support letting people feel heard and allowing others to share their experiences too Those conversations are SO meaningful and will honestly make a bigger impact on facilitating change amongst your patients than just reiterating the diet plan you already printed and put in their post-op binder.

Inconsistencies, Communication, and Lack of Evidence-Based Guidance

One of the biggest issues I see when it comes to caring for bariatric patients is the inconsistencies and communication.

Inconsistencies within the Interdisciplinary Team

If you want to make sure you are effectively communicating with your patients and that they understand and comprehend the things you are telling them that starts with effective communications among the interdisciplinary team members.

I'm a HUGE advocate for an interdisciplinary approach to treating obesity and for making sure our patients have successful outcomes. This means care is comprehensive and includes surgeons, nurses/nurse practitioners, bariatric oordinators, dietitians, therapists, exercise physiologists/trainers, etc. It real- y does take a village.

ut in that village, everyone has their own role to play, and that role should nhance and support the other roles amongst the team.

One of the biggest issues I see is miscommunication and disagreements mongst the bariatric team, which always trickles down to the patient.

or example, I often see surgeons, nurses, and dietitians within the same center iving different instructions and guidelines to the patient.

I'm so confused. My dietitian told me to take bariatric vitamins, but my sur- eon said Flintstones and over-the-counter ones were fine."

My dietitian said I need to increase my fiber and suggested adding more hole grains, but my surgeon told me I need to be keto and not eat any carbs, o I'm not really sure what I'm supposed to do."

My surgeon told me he wants me at 1,000 calories per day, but my dietitian old me not to worry about the calories and focus more on my protein."

My dietitian told me I'm doing a great job, but then the nurse practitioner eighed me and told me I need to cut back and have liquids again."

All real things patients have said to me. No wonder they're confused. It's SO mportant that the entire team is not only on the same page with what the rec- mmendations are, but that they respect the role of each person on their team.

know I'm biased here, but I really feel it's inappropriate for anyone besides he dietitian to be giving nutrition advice. Just like a dietitian shouldn't be ad- ising on which surgery to choose or which medication to take, surgeons and urses shouldn't be telling patients what to eat or what to cut out without first discussing it with the dietitian.

This confuses and overwhelms patients, not to mention creates a pretty big ri in the trust they have within their care team. Many are less likely to reach ou for support or for help when they need it if they don't trust the informatio they are being given because they keep hearing different things from differer people.

<u>Inconsistencies within the Field of Bariatrics as a Whole</u>

I think perhaps one of the most frustrating (and confusing) things is the va iability within the field of bariatrics as a whole. I think what is SO confusin to bariatric patients, and to those deciding whether or not to have surgery, i why the post-op guidelines, diet, and lifestyle requirements are different fro bariatric center to bariatric center.

Despite all the evidence-based research, the ASMBS guidelines, and everythin we have learned about obesity care as a whole, it is WILD to me that there sti is no standardization amongst bariatric centers when it comes to the post-o diet recommendations and instructions. The only thing I see that is universa ly the same and consistent amongst bariatric centers is the following:

- Recommending 60 grams of protein
- Recommending 64 ounces of fluid
- Recommending the liquid/puréed/soft food progression stages

And even amongst these things, there is still variation. I had someone recentl tell me that, until she came to work with me, she never even knew about th recommendation of 60 grams of protein per day. Her center had an "intuitiv eating" approach and didn't give patients target ranges for any nutrients. An you all know how I feel about intuitive eating for bariatric patients!

Unfortunately, each bariatric center has their own philosophies and approac es to weight loss surgery. I'm not saying one approach is wrong and one is right (okay, who am I kidding, there ARE some approaches I think are wrong, looking at you intuitive eating WLS centers!), but there has got to be better standardization across the board.

Lack of Evidence-Based Guidance

With the lack of standardization in philosophies to approaching WLS unfortunately comes too many recommendations that simply are not evidence based. The most common recommendations I see being given from bariatric surgeons, dietitians, and practitioners that, in my opinion, are simply unethical, include the following:

- Don't ever eat over 1,000 calories per day for life
- No carbs/no fruit for life
- Suggestions to "go back to liquids" to "get the scale moving"
- Don't work out, because it will impact your progress on the scale
- Don't work out, because you will be hungrier, and we don't want you eating more
- At least one or two of your meals every day for the rest of your life should be a protein shake

Pardon my French, but all of the above recommendations are complete BS. Sounds more like poor advice given by diet-culture vultures than advice given by your clinical bariatric team. But unfortunately, these are very common recommendations that are given at weight loss surgery centers. They are not evidence based; they are not realistic; they are not healthy; and they confuse the absolute heck out of your clients, especially those who are working so hard to get out of the diet-culture mentality.

It's absolutely wild to me that there are so many WLS clinics that discourage exercise. If your surgeon or dietitian tells you not to exercise, because it will make you weigh more or make you hungrier, throw this book at them as you storm out of their office and go get yourself a new care team. Okay, maybe don't throw things at them, but certainly consider going somewhere else for your post-op care.

It's truly unethical for your care team to worry more about your weight and your BMI than your overall health. Because here's the thing: if you are working out and moving your body, sure, you might see slower weight loss if you are maintaining or building muscle mass, and you likely will be hungrier after working out; HOWEVER, that's not a bad thing! When you work out and maintain/build muscle, you are healthier and more likely to have a higher BMR, which is shown to be best for long-term sustainable weight loss results. If your team only cares about seeing the lowest number possible at the expense of your health, it's time to search for new practitioners in your area who will take better care of you.

The same goes if your team is discouraging you from slowly increasing your calories long term. Any surgical team whose philosophy is to keep calories under 1,000 per day long term and who suggests you cut out all food and go on a "pouch reset" to "get the scale moving" belongs in the same category as the surgical teams who discourage exercise.

Pouch resets are a really common, really dangerous practice amongst the bariatric community. Basically, a pouch reset is when a bariatric patient who has advanced back to solid foods goes back to a full-liquid diet in hopes to get the scale moving again when they are stalled or regaining. The idea is it will reset your thinking, get you "back on track," and "reset" your pouch, making you feel that tight restriction again you experienced immediately post-op.

Pouch resets are by far the WORST trend we have in the bariatric community. And I understand why patients do them: they see others doing them, and sometimes eating nothing at all is easier than dealing with your impaired relationship with food. Also, the idea of losing weight quickly is appealing; I get it.

But for surgeons and dietitians to actually recommend this? How in the world are we supposed to expect bariatric patients to create healthy habits if their care teams are the ones distorting their idea of what a healthy relationship with food and weight loss should be? And no, pouch resets do NOT work. Sure, you might lose a few pounds while doing it, but drinking liquids isn't sustainable; and as soon as you eat again, you are going to gain all the weight back, just like with every other fad diet you've ever done. And no, it does not "shrink" or "reset" your pouch. If you have nothing but liquids for one to two weeks, of course you're going to feel that fullness once you start to eat again, because you've just starved yourself for a few weeks. It doesn't mean anything has changed anatomically or mentally.

Insurance Coverage & Medical Tourism

Another major gap in the system is the constraints laid out by insurance companies. Cost and insurance in the US plays a major role in the type of support that's provided, if people are able to receive surgery at all.

Financial concerns are a huge barrier to being able to receive support. It's especially frustrating when the insurance companies are the ones that dictate what the patient needs to complete in order to qualify for surgery.

When I was going through the pre-op stages, I was very fortunate to have good insurance that covered the majority of the costs at the time. However, per my insurance company, I needed six consecutive monthly nutrition visits before I could get approval. The caveat here was that my insurance plan only would cover a maximum of three nutrition visits within one year's time. So three of those sessions I had to pay for out of pocket at $250 per appointment. As a very broke college student, that was quite the burden to figure out on top of all the co-pays for the 20-some-odd appointments I had that year.

Luckily, my surgery was in December, so by January, my insurance kicked in, and I was able to make it to post-op nutrition visits right after surgery. But had timing not been on my side, I definitely wouldn't have been able to go to those appointments afterwards; and let me tell you, I needed them

Because insurance is such a hassle and costs for surgery here in the US ar quite high (upwards of $25,000 out of pocket on average[134]), many people see what's called **medical tourism**, which means going outside of the US to re ceive their weight loss surgery at a lesser cost. One of the most common loca tion where weight loss surgery operations are sought out is in Mexico, wher the cost of surgery, care, food, and stay is usually around $4,000 or so.

Many of these surgical centers do offer great surgical care, and in many sce narios, there are US board-certified surgeons performing these surgeries. Bu unfortunately, when you have surgery in Mexico, there is next to no suppor or pre- or post-op care and education. You usually don't receive any nutritio guidance at all. The other problem is that if you choose to have surgery ou side of the US, many doctors within the US will not treat you in the event you have complications once you return. So unfortunately, oftentimes, people ar not able to find a bariatric surgeon once they return who will oversee thei medical care.

Cultural Competencies & Awareness

Another area where I see so many opportunities for improvement to provid ing better pre- and post-op care is in making sure that the interdisciplinary team is sensitive and understanding of different cultures, faiths, tradition and potential barriers to being able to fully make the changes necessary.

I dive into this in much greater detail in Chapter 14, but ultimately, what see from a dietitian perspective is a generally poor understanding of how to counsel and educate people of various backgrounds and cultures. And to be totally honest, even though I'm aware of how important it is to be giving my

[134] "Average Cost of Gastric Bypass Surgery," "Weight Loss Surgeries: Gastric Bypass" of Obesity Coverage website, accessed on July 16, 2023, https://www.obesitycoverage.com/insurance-and-costs/how-much/average-laparoscopic-gastric-bypass-prices.

lients culturally relevant and appropriate suggestions, I'm not always sure 'hat those suggestions should look like.

.ny RD can tell you that our education is severely lacking when it comes) cultural awareness. Coming from a field that is dominated by White fe-ıales, most of us have only had one class in all of our schooling on cultural ompetence and awareness, if we're lucky enough. I received only a one-hour resentation in my dietetic internships about accommodating different cul-ıres. Luckily, I've since sought out my own education, but unfortunately, not veryone does.

here is a huge issue when people from different cultural backgrounds receive ariatric nutrition counseling. So often, they are told to just stop eating their ultural foods and eat foreign food items instead. Not only is this completely ısensitive and unrealistic, it's also completely unnecessary. This lack of un-erstanding and awareness also tends to lead to mistrust of bariatric providers, nd oftentimes, these patients are less likely to seek out help or support when ıey need it.

:mpathy- and Patient-Centered Care

'm a firm believer that, as healthcare providers, we should ALWAYS be taking n individualized and patient-centered care approach. How can we expect to ıake bariatric surgery a "one-size-fits-all" process when obesity itself is such complex and nuanced disease?

o many bariatric patients come to me and feel like they are just another num-er coming through the revolving door at their center. They tell me they some-imes feel judged, and they often feel misunderstood or dismissed. They feel ike they aren't being heard when they have concerns or questions, or they feel ike no one on their bariatric team is able or willing to individualize their plan o accommodate and fit their needs.

If you are a patient and have felt this way, I will tell you what I tell my client you deserve to be an active participant in the care you are receiving. Bein told what to do or what to follow without any accommodations made whe you express your concerns, doubts, or hesitations isn't okay. If you vocalize struggle you are having and are told to "just follow the diet," "just go back t liquids," or that you should "probably just lower your calories," that is such one-size-fits-all approach. Everyone's needs are unique, and they deserve t be treated as such.

When I was still working full time as a clinical dietitian, I applied for some lo cal bariatric dietitian positions. I applied to work at a local weight loss surger center in their full-time RD position with a surgeon who is very well-know well-respected, and has been operating and caring for WLS patients for ove 30 years. Turns out, longer doesn't mean better, and that was very telling b his archaic protocol.

After interviewing, I landed the job. The surgeon loved the idea of havin a bariatric patient who was also a dietitian giving nutrition education. Th problem is, and this a common problem at a lot of centers, the surgeon di tates what the dietitian is and is not allowed to say (this goes back to what was saying before about discrepancies amongst the clinical team).

He was shocked when I turned down the job. I was kind of shocked I turned i down too. At the time, I was pretty miserable working my long-term-care jol and I so badly wanted to work with bariatric patients. But after I interviewe I knew there was no way I could work for this center in good conscience.

This particular surgeon stood by his philosophy that every patient should sta under 1,000 calories per day for life. He said, and I quote, "As soon as we se their weight start to trickle up, or we see they are eating upwards of 1,20 calories a day, we put them on phentermine. No ifs, ands, or buts. They don' have a choice."

Do you ever have those moments when you have to actively remind yoursel o control your facial expressions? That was me at that moment. I was actively rying to hide my disgust.

Now listen, you all know I'm all for the use of anti-obesity medications when ndicated. But only if the patient is open to it! It was also wild to me to see hat he only cared about weight, not overall health or body composition. We know that almost no one stays at their lowest weight, and I think shaming and forcing people to try to by any means necessary is so not okay.

As a dietitian who would be working for this man, I would have to back his approach and follow his philosophy of educating patients to only eat 1,000 calories per day. Ethically, I just could not do that. So I turned the job down.

I guess things still worked out okay for me though, and I'm here to tell the tale to all of you fine people. Ironically enough, a few months after that interview, once I went full time in my own business, I was working with a client who was actually a patient of this surgeon.

She was struggling with regain and made the choice to no longer go back to her surgeon for the exact reasons I chose not to work for him. He wanted to put her on phentermine, and that wasn't what she wanted. He also wanted her to significantly reduce her calories to unhealthy levels for her based on her height and weight and activity level. So she walked away. Instead, she used my approach of individualized care, empathy, and understanding; got her regain under control; and proceeded to run a 5k that summer.

The point here is that a little bit of empathy and understanding can go a long way. And individualizing care will always be better for the patient. Period.

Playing Devil's Advocate

I've had more conversations with bariatric colleagues than I can count, and I've been in healthcare long enough to know that sometimes a practitioner's love for patient care and dedication to their patients just isn't enough for them to be able to provide them with the support and care they would like to give.

Our healthcare providers are chronically overworked, understaffed, and underpaid. It's SO frustrating when, as a practitioner, you so badly want to be able to sit with your patients for as long as it takes to help them feel supported and to go above and beyond. But when most practitioners are seeing upwards of 8–16 patients per day (yes, some are literally expected to care for that many during an 8-hour shift in their outpatient bariatric offices), how in the world are they supposed to give their patients the support and one-on-one time they truly need?

It's so hard to get to truly know people and to be able to give them the hand-holding through this process they so badly need and deserve.

Our healthcare system is truly stacked against us. This for-profit system is driving healthcare providers into the ground. And when everything is dictated by insurance, and you have to bill someone for a 30-minute session, you truly can't spend the hour with them that is really needed to make sure they understand what you're teaching them.

It's really not an ideal system or process for anyone.

My Hope for the Future

While everyone's experiences with surgical care varies, universally, it seems most bariatric patients feel they need more care, and most WLS practitioners feel they need more time to provide that care. It's my hope that with ongoing education, awareness, and understanding, we can continue to improve the patient care experience. I'm not sure what the answer is, but I do know we have so many areas we can work on improving. Bariatrics continues to be a growing and evolving field, and bariatrics isn't going anywhere anytime soon. I hope as a field, we can continue to adapt and accommodate ALL our patients, so veryone has the best chances at having a successful surgery experience.

nd to every bariatric patient reading this—be your own advocate. It is not our responsibility as the patient to fix the broken pieces of our healthcare ystem. And while those of us in the medical field do our best to try and make hanges so future patients' experiences can be better, you still deserve support ow.

o learn more about how to advocate for yourself, how to find a Bariatric enter of Excellence, and how to find a primary care physician who is double board-certified in obesity medicine, head to www.thesleeveddietitian.com/asy for more resources and ways to find support.

Bite-Sized Recap

- When it comes to bariatric care and support, many patients might fe misunderstood, under-supported, or even confused with the thing that are being asked of them.
- Bariatrics patients often need more support than their clinicians an surgical centers are able to provide.
- There is generally much more support for bariatric patients who ar pre-op than those who are post-op.
- Improving lines of communication amongst the interdisciplinary tean will likely help with inconsistencies in the care received, making for better patient experience.
- More education including cultural competencies and awareness of nu anced situations can help the interdisciplinary team better understan and empathize with their patients.
- Insurance coverage and costs continue to be a barrier to surgery.
- Those who seek medical tourism need and deserve better suppor upon return to the States.
- Most bariatric professionals want all of these things for their patient too. However, healthcare providers are chronically overworked, ur derstaffed, and underpaid, making it incredibly difficult to close thes gaps.
- While everyone's experience with surgical care varies, universally, i seems most bariatric patients feel they need more care, and most WL practitioners feel they need more time to provide that care. Ongoin education, awareness, and understanding can continue to improve th patient care experience.

For journal prompts and resources related to this chapter be sure to head to www thesleeveddietitian.com/easy.

Chapter 16
The Grief That Comes Along with Change

;rief

;ri:f/

oun

. deep sorrow, especially caused by someone's loss

She was overcome with grief."

. trouble or annoyance

Dealing with other people's opinions was too much grief."

he Old Me

hey say there are five stages of grief: denial, anger, bargaining, depression, nd acceptance.

or a long time, I denied the fact that I had to let parts of myself and my festyle go to make my goals happen on this journey—to actually make the hanges I needed to in order to have surgery and be successful at it. Not just or the sake of weight loss, but to live the life I'd always wanted to. I denied vhat was underneath all of my weight struggles.

was angry at times. I would think about past, younger versions of myself and eel absolute rage towards her. *How could you let us get here? Why did you let s get so big?* I was angry with her for making me feel backed up against the vall with no other option but to have surgery. And I felt angry with her when ooking back on all the years and experiences we missed out on: never going n dates or hanging out with friends, always staying on the sidelines of our wn life. I spent a lot of time resenting her for that.

I tried bargaining with myself. In the pre-op stages, I'd say to myself, *Oka Jamie, if you can just lose 20 pounds. in the next six months, you can cancel yo surgery*. I told myself if I could just "prove" I could do it "on my own," the I wouldn't have to let go and take the leap to have surgery. *If you just try o more time, maybe it will work out this time,* I thought.

And I spent a lot of time being sad and depressed, thinking back to past ve sions of myself. I'm sad for her. For us. And everything we missed out on an had to deal with. Looking back at pictures of me at my heaviest, seeing ho sad I was behind the fake smile, makes me want to cry still to this day.

But I've finally accepted that the "old me" did what she could. I can resent he all I want, for the things she couldn't do or wasn't strong enough to handle. Bu the truth is, she was so much stronger than I ever gave her credit for. Becaus she got me here. I would not be the person I am today without honoring an accepting the old versions of myself.

And it's okay that I'm not who I used to be anymore. It's okay that I've had t let parts of myself go to become who I am now.

When I post old pictures or talk about my journey, I often refer to pre-surger Jamie as the "old me." I still have a complicated relationship with her. Som days, I'm still angry at her. Some days, I'm still sad for her. Some days, I eve miss her and all her old coping mechanisms, habits, and routines. And whil obviously, there are parts of me that are still the same—I like to think my in tegrity, kindness, and empathy for others has never faltered—the truth is, I an different. I have changed. I have become the person I always wanted to be an dreamed of being.

I'm not the same person. I've grown and evolved into an entirely differen human being. There was no way I could have bypassed these stages of grief o this journey, even if I wanted to.

Grieving Your Old Life and Lifestyle

In the years of therapy, over six months of pre-op counseling, and more than 27 different pre-op appointments, not once did anyone tell me I would experience grief on this journey. You're told to prepare and get ready for your new life, but no one ever prepares you for the life you lose in the process.

During support groups in my T.R.I.B.E® Membership Program, grief comes up often. So much so, I hired a therapist this last year to specifically lead grief support groups. Now of course, we talk about and honor "true" losses in the sense of death, because dealing with losing a loved one on this journey can be absolutely devastating. But we also talk a lot about ambiguous losses.

An ambiguous loss is when you lose someone who remains physically here on this Earth. This might mean grieving a person who is alive and well but no longer a part of your life. Ambiguous losses usually are not accompanied by closure, which makes them harder to wrap our heads around.

And sometimes, what you lose is yourself and your old lifestyle. Sometimes it's not even a person. Rather, it's food or that coping skill you used to lean on.

If you find yourself sad after surgery, and you weren't expecting it, know that you may simply be grieving. It's okay to miss food. It's okay to cry because you can't eat the way you used to. It's okay if you cry because you can't eat the same foods as your family or friends at a party or picnic. You can grieve the ways you used to eat food socially. You're allowed to miss your old lifestyle, even if you know it wasn't a healthy one for you.

You're allowed to grieve the way you used to look. It's okay if you don't feel at home in your new body. If you feel a sense of "homesickness" or "longing," it may just be that you are missing the parts of you that aren't there anymore. Or missing what you used to see in the mirror. Because not everyone who has WLS was unhappy with their lifestyle or their appearance before surgery. It's done for more than cosmetic reasons. And if you don't recognize yourself now, that's valid.

And you may be grieving other heavy things too. Whatever your grief is, it's valid. It's not silly.

So try to be a bit gentler with yourself than you've been in the past. Even if your old lifestyle or old coping mechanisms don't serve you anymore, they served their purpose at one point in time. Whether it was emotional eating, binging, or something else, those things once kept you safe from something, even if it was just you protecting yourself from your own feelings.

Grief is ongoing, and getting to a point of acceptance takes time.

Grieving the People Who Walk Away and Whom You Walk Away From

Another thing you may hear about embarking on this journey is that your relationships, friendships, and family dynamics might suffer. You may think, *Oh, that will never happen to me. The people in my life support me unconditionally.* And for some of you, that may be true. I can honestly say that I am truly fortunate and blessed that the majority of people in my life do support me through and through. But even still, that doesn't mean I haven't lost people along the way. Some have walked away from me, others I have walked away from.

Romantic Relationships

In 2022, a research study from the University of Pittsburgh looked at data from 1,441 bariatric patients and found that married bariatric patients were twice as likely to get divorced compared to the general population. On the same token though, interestingly enough, they also found that non-married bariatric patients were also 50% more likely to get married after surgery.[135]

[135] Wendy King et al., "Changes in Marital Status Following Roux-en-Y Gastric Bypass and Sleeve Gas-

Unfortunately, divorce and separation is common after weight loss surgery. here are lots of factors that might play into this. It's a big deal when someone oses an extreme amount of weight. Sometimes, this leaves partners feeling nferior or insecure. Sometimes, the person who lost the weight doesn't feel upported or realizes they were settling for certain treatment or a certain life-tyle before their self-worth increased. There are so many nuances here.

'm so fortunate to have an incredible husband who's been supportive, but I've nown many other people who haven't had the same level of support from heir partner. My relationship with my husband has also really opened my yes as to how weight in relationships is perceived by the general public.

People are always so surprised to learn I started dating my husband back in 2014, three years before my weight loss surgery. He was with me when I was bigger and was also with me as I continued to gain weight. And the comments received from people in my own life when I started dating him were really quite baffling.

You see, my husband has never struggled with his weight. He's lean and fit and what society would deem as "conventionally attractive." When I started dating him, some of the comments I received were as follows:

"Wow, that's your boyfriend?"

"Wait, you're dating him? He's actually cute!"

"Oh, I'm surprised; he's good looking. That's not who I pictured you with."

It's wild, because these comments came from friends and family alike, and it's as if it genuinely didn't occur to them that this was hurtful to me.

---

rectomy: A US Multicenter Prospective Cohort Study," Annals of Surgery Open 3, no. 3 (September 2022): 182, https://journals.lww.com/aosopen/Fulltext/2022/09000/Changes_in_Marital_Status_Following_Roux_en_Y.8.aspx#JCL-P-12.

Weight shouldn't matter when it comes to relationships. But it does. Every one's attracted to different body types (and apparently, it was just completel unbelievable that my "hot" boyfriend was attracted to me at the time). Bu weight plays an even bigger role in relationships when it comes to dynamic roles, needs, confidence, and self-worth.

I have had many friends in this community finally reach their healthiest weigh and start to feel like their happiest and most authentic selves, only to be face with their spouse leaving them or with the tough decision to walk away fron their partner. I can't imagine what that level of grief feels like, but I'm holdin space and sending love to everyone in our community who has gone throug this.

Friendships & Family Dynamics

Unfortunately, friendships and family relationships are not excluded from th list of losses that sometimes occur on this journey.

In many situations, friends and family aren't supportive of your decision to have surgery. They will often say things like this:

"Well, have you tried dieting and exercising?"

"Are you sure you need that? You're not even that big."

"I think you can do it on your own."

"Oh, I know someone who had surgery. They gained all their weight back."

"You don't need surgery. You're beautiful just the way you are."

"You should just do it naturally, like I did."

You always take the easy way out and cut corners. If you worked harder, you ould lose weight."

lot of these comments are unsolicited, unhelpful, backhanded, and overall nsupportive. They can really make an already lonely experience feel even ıore isolating. And the comments usually don't stop there.

Iany people also experience unsolicited, unhelpful, backhanded, and even ısulting comments after surgery too:

OMG, how much weight have you lost?/How much do you weigh now?"

You're not going to keep losing are you? You're too skinny. You should stop ow."

That's all you're going to eat?"

Are you sure you should be eating that?"

Can you really eat all of that?"

Vhile I haven't experienced all of these comments, I've experienced a great eal of them, and the others are comments many of my clients tell me they've eceived. It's odd. For some reason, some people see you've had surgery, or ave lost a lot of weight, and suddenly forget all their manners regarding what s and isn't okay to ask someone or comment on.

Vhen I was about five months post-op or so, I went to visit my grandmother, vho I had a troubled relationship with. My entire life, she always had something negative to say. But I thought, *Maybe this time she'll be proud of me.* I vas down about 50 pounds., and I thought for sure, this time, she would have omething positive to say. But I was wrong.

She looked at me and said, with a scolding look on her face, "What have yo been doing? Your legs are even bigger now than they were before! You reall need to stop working out so much; it's just making your legs bigger." And sh didn't stop there. "And I would have thought with the weight loss your acn would have cleared up by now," she added.

You literally can't make this shit up.

It's important to note that, while direct and outward comments like these ca be really hurtful, sometimes the silence from those around us is even worse.

This seems to happen a lot within friendships. Many people have told me the lost their best friends along this journey—friends who also struggled wit their weight and disagreed with them for having surgery, friends who weren able to be supportive due to their own struggles, or friends who just plain wer en't able to be there for them.

It's not always the weight loss itself that imposes on your friendships. Some times when people see you growing, changing, and leveling up in your life, can make them feel as if they are falling behind. And in some cases, even if it subconscious and not intentional, some people prefer it when we aren't doin as well as they are, because it makes them feel better about themselves. Whe they recognize you doing better and rising up, sometimes scarcity and fear ca show up within them.

I like to see the good in people and believe that most don't mean to inflict pai on those they love. But some people simply aren't able to give us what we need That's not their fault, and it's not yours either. Some people get so used to yo being the quiet friend (or maybe playing the role of the "funny, fat" friend that when you are no longer the quiet sidekick, it makes them feel discomfort And honestly? That has nothing to do with us.

I say it all the time, but you are the only one responsible for your triggers

So if your success or change triggers something within someone else, that is their issue and their issue alone. You are not responsible for how your circumstances make them feel. And if someone makes you feel less than or triggers insecurities within you, it's your job to figure out what boundaries you need to set and maintain.

You certainly don't have to cut people out of your life who you love. Not all disagreements or unsupportive moments result in walking away from one another. But if someone in your life who you love isn't supporting you, showing up for you, or being the person you need them to be, it's up to you to figure out what boundaries you need to set.

Maybe that starts with setting your own boundaries first. Maybe that means setting a boundary to not share certain wins with certain people who aren't willing or able to celebrate them with you. Or maybe, to people in your life who continue to say hurtful or passive-aggressive things, that means saying, "Hey, I'd appreciate it if you didn't make comments about my body or my food choices."

And if they can't respect those boundaries, then it's up to you to decide in what ways you allow those people to be a part of your life, if at all.

I've had people say such hurtful things to me, especially after my weight loss surgery. And even though I've forgiven them, for my own well-being, I simply just can't have them in my life anymore. It doesn't mean I don't miss them or no longer love them; it just means I can't allow myself to continue to be hurt by them. And even if cutting toxic relationships out of your life happens on your terms, you're still allowed to be sad about it and grieve it.

Some people simply don't know how to be the person you need them to be. And unfortunately, sometimes it takes a change as massive as weight loss surgery to realize that.

"Wow, You've Changed."

Why yes, yes I have. Thank you so much for noticing.

No one goes through weight loss surgery with the goal in mind to stay the same. Whether you realize it or not, you're going to change more than just your body size. You cannot possibly go through this and come out on the other side exactly the same as you were before.

And hopefully, the changes that happen are mostly positive. Nothing is ever perfect, but hopefully, with everything you've lost along the way, you've gained something twice as meaningful and valuable.

People sling the phrase "You've changed" in your face after surgery like it's an insult. The hard truth is that not everyone is going to like you or support you once you do start to go through these changes. That's okay. Not everyone has to. But you don't have to stick around people who continue to make you feel bad about all the progress you've made. Don't let anyone mistake your happiness and confidence for arrogance. You and I both know that's not the case.

You're always going to be the villain in someone else's story. That's okay. No one but you gets to walk in your shoes or live the life you do. So if losing weight, gaining confidence, and changing and shifting your life priorities makes other people uncomfortable or causes them to no longer "like" you—well, that's not your responsibility, babe. What other people think of you is not your burden to carry.

Those who love and support you unconditionally will be by your side no matter your size. They will lift you up and cheer you on as you strive for new goals and become happier and healthier. And anyone who doesn't does not deserve a seat at your table anyway. And just know, there is a whole bariatric community out here ready to support you and uplift you in ways other people in your life never can.

Bite-Sized Recap

- Grief may be an unanticipated experience both before and after weight loss surgery.
- Many people grieve their old lifestyle, habits, and body. Although bariatric surgery usually yields a desired change, it doesn't mean that there isn't some sadness and grief associated with the habits and lifestyle you must leave behind in order to pursue new dreams and goals.
- You may have to grieve romantic relationships after surgery.
- Friendships and family relationships are not excluded from the list of losses that sometimes occur on this journey.
- It's not always the weight loss itself that imposes on your friendships and relationships. Sometimes, when people see you growing, changing, and leveling up in your life, it can make them feel as if they are falling behind which can ultimately shift the dynamics of your relationship, forcing it to change.
- No one goes through weight loss surgery with the goal in mind to stay the same. Whether you realize it or not, you're going to change more than just your body size. You cannot possibly go through this and come out on the other side exactly the same as you were before.

For journal prompts and resources related to this chapter be sure to head to <u>www.thesleeveddietitian.com/easy</u>.

Chapter 17
The Importance of Community on Your Journey

com·mu·ni·ty
/kəmyoonədē/
noun
1. a group of people living in the same place or having a particular character-istic in common
"the bariatric community"
2. a feeling of fellowship with others, as a result of sharing common beliefs, interests, and goals
"the sense of community that organized religion can provide"

The Community I Craved

It's hard to describe the level of isolation I felt when starting my bariatric journey. As badly as I wanted the surgery—knowing, in my heart, I needed it if wanted to live a long, healthy, and fulfilling life—I was also terrified. And I had never met anyone in my life who had walked this path and had the surgery. had no one to talk to about it who understood what I was feeling and going through.

Additionally, during my six month pre-op stage, leading up to the surgery, was working my dietetic internship and surrounded by dietitians who lived in much smaller bodies than mine. This added to how utterly alone I felt. I already felt judged by them, and I knew some of them didn't support or "agree" with bariatrics.

ther than my immediate family and boyfriend (now husband), I chose not to iare my impending surgery with anyone. I felt like a hypocrite of a soon-to-e dietitian for not being able to do it "on my own." And after so many failed iet attempts, I was afraid to be a failure again, unable to actually lose the eight. So I told no one.

arrying around this secret pushed me into further isolation. In my loneliess, I started seeking support on social media. I created a private Instagram :count and joined private Facebook pages, where I lurked and watched other eople's journeys.

/hile it was nice to chat with people on social media and hear their experiices, I found it ultimately sparked more anxiety than it reduced, especially n Facebook. I would get completely absorbed in threads created by someone osting an innocent question or a win who was met with criticism, bashing, id shaming, rather than support or congratulations. Plus, the nutrition exert in me had a real problem with all the misinformation I saw regarding ost-op diets and lifestyle changes.

noticed a clear difference between the support I received on Facebook versus istagram. Some toxic diet culture and misinformation still existed there, but seemed to be far less present. I started following people who truly inspired ie. (Shout out to @skinnyminipaige and @recreatingnicole for being the first eople I ever looked up to on this journey!)

ı 2018, I signed up to go to a local, in-person meetup hosted by Nicole from)recreatingnicole. Given that this took place when I was just three weeks ost-op, I was still brand new to surgery and extremely nervous. I didn't know hat to expect.

Ve all met at a restaurant and sat down to have dinner together, and I can onestly say that going was the best thing I could have done on my personal ›urney. It changed the trajectory of my post-op journey. I sat down at a tale with women who showed me nothing but genuine kindness, support, and love. And the girl I sat directly next to (who is also named Nicole), to this da is still one of my closest friends and biggest supporters.

Those women—Nicole (both Nicoles!), Sara, Colleen, Rae, Jess, and Cour ney—welcomed me, supported me, and showed me what it meant to have community behind me. They made me feel less alone and were the first peop to tell me I could be successful.

So if you're reading this, thank you. I don't know if you'll ever know how muc this still means to me.

Complexities of the Bariatric Community

Those in your corner should support you, lift you up, and cheer you on. The should be honest and genuine with you, holding you accountable and givin you tough love when you need it, just as much as they should hold space fc you and validate your feelings. They should celebrate you, help you, guide yo and uplift you. They should make you feel included, wanted, and important- because you are.

It's important to surround yourself with a community that works for you. Fc some that might mean one or two close friends, for others that might mea connecting with dozens of like-minded individuals, in person or on the ir ternet. Regardless of the type of community you thrive in, your communit should not make you feel inferior, left out, or dismissed. It should not leav you feeling disrespected or invalidated. The support your people offer shoul not be conditional. Your community should not spark comparison or compe tition and should not leave you feeling anything but important, seen, hear and understood.

I share this because I sometimes worry about the ways the bariatric commu nity has shifted in its messaging over time. For those who may not know, ther is a *very* large bariatric community on social media—primarily Facebook, Ir stagram, and TikTok. Instagram is the main community I partake in, both professionally and personally. It's simultaneously one of the most beautiful and encouraging spaces to be in and one of the most toxic. I do believe the positives of it truly outweigh the negatives, and I love this community with my whole heart. But I think it's important to bring to light some of its issues, because how are we ever supposed to make headway with advocacy if we are too busy fighting each other?

While the vast majority of weight loss surgery accounts truly exist to support, encourage, and make friends, some toxic messaging still comes through. As both a professional and patient in the space, I believe there are many messages in the bariatric Instagram community that can unintentionally harm its members. Below, you'll find a table of these concerns.

Disclaimer: This is my personal opinion and interpretation of some of the messaging taking place in the bariatric community on Instagram and social media. You may not see or experience it the way I do or the way I see my clients experiencing it, and that's okay. These mentions are not intended to single out any one person or platform but, rather, to bring awareness to these trends and messages as a whole.

Potentially Toxic Recurring Themes within the WLS Social Media Communities

Message	How It Looks and Why It May Be Harmful
Comparison	People often look to their peers in this community for support and inspiration, and sometimes this can feed into the comparison game—especially when someone is losing weight more quickly, hitting different goals, etc.

Disordered Eating Behavior	Certain well-meaning trends can end up triggering disordered eating behavior. Before-and-after pictures of food eaten on one's plate is a particularly harmful trend, as it can unintentionally create a competitive mindset of seeing "who can eat the least amount." Pouch resets are another toxic trend.
Toxic Positivity	Only seeing the "good" parts of someone's journey or their wins—especially through a filtered lens—perpetuates the idea that you must be positive all the time on this journey, and if you're not, you must be doing something wrong. This doesn't often leave room for validating struggles, which is crucial for this community. Despite people being as real and honest as they can be online, these are still only snippets and highlight reels of someone's life. You will never see the whole picture.
Food Police	Many times in the WLS community, when you share a picture of your post-op meal or food, you are met with comments like "Oh, that's way too much food," "I could never eat all that," "You aren't supposed to eat that," etc.
Misinformation	Inaccurate information is freely given and shared daily. And often, the content creator doesn't even know it's misinformation. This has the potential to greatly influence someone's decision-making after surgery in a very negative way.

I don't believe these issues and trends are unique to the bariatric community; they exist as some of the downfalls of social media as a whole. However, with the bariatric community being as small as it is—as well as being as vulnerable as it is due to lack of support, resources, and community—these things have more potential to cause real harm.

The bariatric journey is not a competition to see who lost the most weight or who can eat the least, nor is it a competition to see who can gain the most followers or post the prettiest posed photo. But that's what it feels like some days.

The bariatric community has become a marketing target from both large brands and the influencers who represent them. Many large supplement companies have realized the vast amount of bariatric patients on Instagram and have hired the larger influencer accounts in the space. As a member of the community, it can be easy to feel like you are constantly being sold something or marketed to, which can also start to make connections feel less genuine and more conditional—based on your purchase, your like, or your follow.

I don't want to run the risk of sounding hypocritical, because I too market myself and my career through social media, and I think everyone has the right to create a business or represent a business and get paid for it. I have absolutely zero problem with people making an income off their social presence and the work they do. The problem comes when people who are not credentialed, or lack the expertise or education to do so, start selling and promoting the things they do.

I've said this before, and I'll say it again: just because someone lost weight does NOT qualify them to be able to help you lose weight. In the bariatric social space, people often go from patient to "coach." Someone will have surgery and start opening up in the community in order to give and receive support; then they lose weight, become more confident, and their account grows, boosting their perceived credibility. People look to them for support and ask them questions. And in time, that patient will label themself a "coach," despite having no training or credentials.

The thing that bothers me most of all is the way the programs of these individuals are often presented. Slowly but surely, I will see them remove their "WLS" tag from their bio, and they no longer present openly as a WLS patient. They stop talking about surgery and start talking about their "coaching" program that promises you results without dieting like "they did." As if it was just that easy.

It's unethical to pitch a service to someone you have no authority or credibility to provide, all the while hiding how you yourself got there in the first place. It actually does NOTHING in terms of advocacy and support for our community and only further stigmatizes it. As a dietitian who went to school for nearly six years to become a credentialed expert, it's so saddening to see people fall into this trap. So many people have come to me after poor experiences with online coaches, resulting in nutrient deficiencies, malnutrition, and more. It's not okay. I understand many do just want to help, but it's easy to fall into the toxic social media trap of forgetting where you came from.

And while I wish I could say that no one actually intends to do harm, I can't. I have been hurt badly in this community. Platforms have stolen my content and the structure of my program, which I worked so hard to build, only to relaunch it as their own. So as you make friendships and lean on people for support in this online community, be a bit guarded. Be mindful of who you invest your time, money, and energy in. And if anyone makes you feel inferior in any way, you have full right and responsibility to yourself to remove them from your feed. Remember, your community should ONLY be supportive and encouraging. If you feel anything but that, you have full permission to walk away.

I'll leave you with this: let your influencers inspire you. But for the love of God, don't let them give you a meal plan.

The Community I've Built around Me

After I attended that first in-person meetup with Nicole, I continued to grow the community around me organically and authentically. The women I met inspired me to keep sharing my surgery journey on social media, and as time went on, I continued to connect with other like-minded people working towards the same goals, or goals similar to mine, online.

I had such beautiful and meaningful conversations with these connections on a daily basis. We celebrated wins with each other, cheered each other on, nd gathered in person at local weight-loss-surgery meetups all throughout Jew England. At each meetup, I met new, beautiful souls I couldn't believe I ad gone my whole life not knowing. The phrase I heard repeatedly at these atherings was "find your tribe." I certainly felt like I had finally found mine.

Vhile building my community, I started my full-time online nutrition busiess, supporting bariatric clients in hitting their goals before and after weight oss surgery. I was, and still am, so grateful for how quickly this business grew. oon, I developed my online membership program, where people could watch elf-paced videos and trainings; receive support; and have access to recipes, vorkouts, and evidence-based resources to guide them on their journey.

But I knew that the thing bariatric patients needed above all else, above even he nutrition and diet support, was the sense of community and belonging. I new this because I *was* them. I've been in their shoes. This led me to launch ny membership program, The Real Insights of Bariatric Eating (also known as T.R.I.B.E.®). Since opening the doors to this support program in 2020, I have welcomed thousands of bariatric patients. And while the resources, materials, and ccess to education it offers has been so powerful—filling the gaps in the postop care system—what's been even more impactful is the community it's created.

As I shared earlier, every month, we host over 40 live support groups for members to meet and talk to one another via Zoom and have meaningful, raw, onest conversations with each other and our credentialed team of leaders all therapists, dietitians, certified trainers, and doctors who have had surgery oo!) We also host in-person T.R.I.B.E.® meetups, facilitating local friendships mongst our members. The people who come to us leave us better than we ound them, because the validation, support, and understanding offered is unnatched.

I created the community and support I didn't have and always wanted. I'm so grateful I found my WLS Instagram friends when I did, and I hope that, by creating a standardized process for post-op support, others on this journey can have it a bit easier than I did. T.R.I.B.E.® was the first membership commu nity of its nature to be brought to fruition, and I'm very proud of it. It's quickl becoming the standard for post-op support and care, as numerous bariatri centers nationwide are sending people to our program.

Recently, a beautiful bariatric babe (who reminded me so much of me when was pre-op) showed up to our support group the night before her surgery. Sh was smiling. She was SO excited for her surgery. We all cheered for her, congrat ulated her, and told her we couldn't wait to hear how she was feeling when sh was in recovery. She told us how grateful she was to not have to do this alone She thanked her bariatric besties in T.R.I.B.E.® for supporting her in the month leading up to this. She said she knew she could do it and would be successful. Sh felt prepared and supported, and most importantly, proud of what she was doing

As I smiled at her through teary eyes, all I could think about was my pre-op self the night before my surgery—alone, crying, afraid, and ashamed. And to think, in such a short time, our community has paved the way for bariatri patients to have a better experience, a better chance at success, and a bette outlook through support and advocacy. This fills my heart with so much joy

This is all I've ever wanted for others. THIS is what I want the bariatric expe rience to look like—not isolating, confusing, and overwhelming. We still have a long way to go in terms of societal understanding and accepting obesity as a disease and bariatrics as a treatment, but we are well on our way.

In the meantime, I'll just be over here, continuing to advocate for our com munity and bariatric patients across the globe. We deserve better. You deserve better. And as we say in the T.R.I.B.E., you can do hard things.

This isn't the easy way out. This journey is anything but easy. But, my God, is it worth it.

Bite-Sized Recap

- Finding a community you can relate to and who understands you is incredibly important and valuable on this journey.
- While the bariatric communities amongst various social media platforms can be incredibly meaningful and valuable, sometimes they can spark comparison and other toxic behaviors.
- Not everyone who has lost weight is qualified to help others lose weight. It's important to be mindful of the resources you are investing in and accepting after surgery.
- Community is going to look different for everyone. For some people, that means being surrounded by many who "get it." For others that might mean having one or two close friends in their inner circle. Whatever community means for you, be sure to seek it out. No one should have to climb this mountain alone.
- No one said it would be easy, This journey is anything but easy. But, my God, is it worth it.

For journal prompts and resources related to this chapter be sure to head to www.thesleeveddietitian.com/easy.

Acknowledgments

I have so much gratitude to all the incredible people in my corner who helped bring my dream of becoming an author to reality. From the time I was a little girl, I used to tell people, "When I grow up, I'm going to be an author." Turns out Little Jamie was manifesting her dreams early!

First and foremost, I want to thank my husband, Steven, and Lilo (our fur baby) for being the best emotional support system a girl could ever ask for. Through the long hours, late nights, and anxieties that come along with putting my story out there, Steven continues to be my shoulder to lean on, and Lilo continues to be my ultimate partner in crime, always laying at my feet while I write (with the occasional interruption of barking at the mailman, of course!).

Thank you to all my friends and family who have been so supportive and encouraging. Especially my mom, who is, and always will be, my biggest supporter. She's been proud of me since day one and continues to be my biggest cheerleader. And I'm so proud of her too, for coming on this bariatric journey with me.

To Rea Frey, Megan Irby, Jackie Hritz, and Alex Holguin from Writeway: thank you from the bottom of my heart for all your support. Without the Writeway team, I can say with confidence that this book wouldn't be here. Or at least, it wouldn't have been here for a very long time. Rea, with your ongoing support, feedback, and encouragement, I was able to bring my dream to life and get this book into the hands of those who needed it most without delaying this resource any longer. Thank you, Rea, for believing in me and my dream and reminding me at every corner that this book was needed and is so important.

Along with the team at Writeway, a special thank you to Dannie Lynn Fountain for introducing me to Rea Frey in the first place. Dannie, you've been such a huge support system to me throughout this journey. Thank you for all you do for me, our T.R.I.B.E.® team, and our community.

To Jaime Mass: without you, The Sleeved Dietitian® and the T.R.I.B.E.® wouldn't be here. Thank you for your unconditional love and ongoing support and coaching over the years. Thank you for making me the entrepreneur I am today and allowing me to grow into the person I was always meant to be. I will never have words to thank you for all you have done for me and my business.

To Cierra, Crystal, Chelsea, Brogan, and the rest of The Sleeved Dietitian® Support Team: thank you for holding down the fort for me while I took the time I needed to keep my head down and get this book done on time. It truly takes a village, and I'm forever grateful to have you as a part of my T.R.I.B.E.®. Thank you for helping me carry out my mission and making sure we are always providing the best of the best for our members.

To my incredible T.R.I.B.E.® Leaders: Marissa, Melissa, Megan, Sam W., Tori, Sam S., Natalie, Mel, Becca, Julie, Laura, Danielle, Alisha, Caleshia, Dannie, Bri, Anna, Mikayla, Chelsea, and Lisa—thank you for all you do for me and for our T.R.I.B.E.®. The T.R.I.B.E.® would not be the incredible space that it is without each and every one of you. You mean the world to me, and I think I can speak on behalf of our entire community when I say thank you for hosting the best support groups and workshops out there.

To all my bariatric friends—there are far too many of you to list, but you know who you are! To those of you who have supported me personally on this journey, lifted me up when I was feeling down, and who have shown me what true friendship looks like, thank you from the bottom of my heart. The impact you have made on me and my own journey is immeasurable. Thank you for providing me a safe space to show up and be unapologetically me.

To all of our T.R.I.B.E.® Members and clients—wow. Just wow. You all blow me away and make me so damn proud each and every day. To see you showing up, putting in the work, and being a support to others on this journey fills my heart with so much joy! Thank you for trusting me to support you. They say if you love what you do you never work a day in your life, and I can tell you from the bottom of my heart, you all make me the happiest dietitian there is. It is a true honor and privilege to support you, and it's a responsibility I do not take lightly and do not take for granted. Thank you for choosing me to come on this journey with you and allowing me to do what I love!

And lastly, to everyone who has ever followed me, subscribed to my emails, liked my posts, read my blogs, purchased any of my products and resources, and engaged with my content—thank you so much!!!! Without you, I wouldn't be here spreading this message to the world. Thank you for being the reason I have the platform I do to be able to continue to do the work that I love. It means so much to me.

And to Little Jamie—to Jamie at 8 years old, who cried because her grandmother made fun of her weight. To 12-year-old Jamie, who was embarrassed she couldn't buy jeans at the mall like the rest of her friends. To 16-year-old Jamie, who was never asked to prom and felt so alone. To 19-year-old Jamie, who struggled immensely with her mental health and was so isolated. To 24-year-old Jamie, who took the leap and had surgery. And to the younger versions of myself at every stage in between—thank you. It might sound strange, and perhaps even egotistical, to thank the past versions of myself, but despite her struggles, she is ultimately who got me here. She never gave up. Somehow she found it in her to keep going and pushing for her dreams. Not a day goes by where I don't thank her for pointing me in the right direction. Because of the action steps my past self has taken, I am here today, sharing my words with all of you. And I will be forever grateful.

Ready to take the next step on your journey?

Join the T.R.I.B.E.®

If you'd like to work together, I would love to invite you to work with me in my signature membership program.

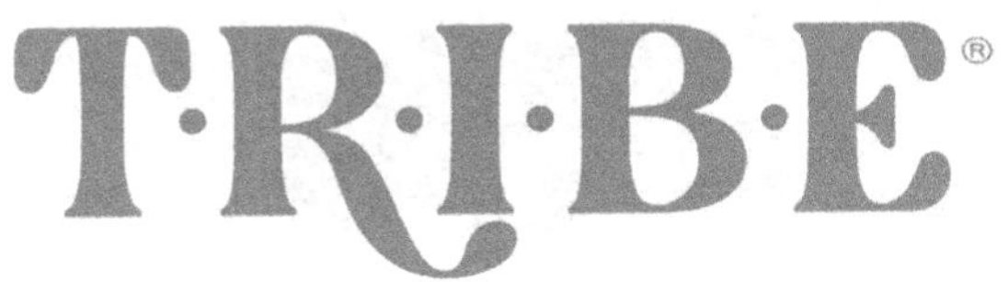

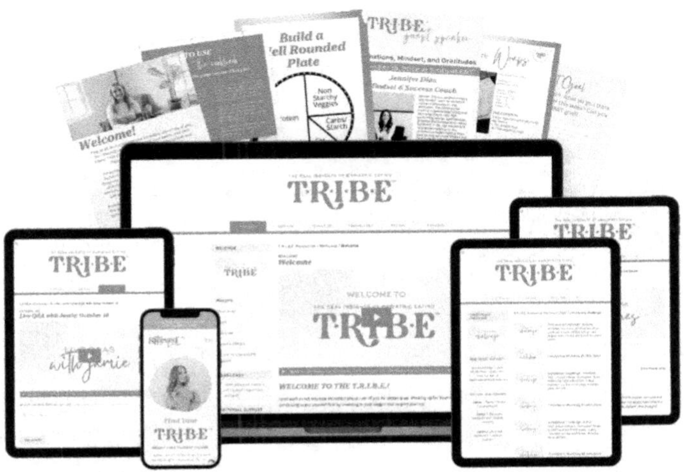

The T.R.I.B.E.® Membership is a self-paced, step-by-step membership for babes pre- and post-weight loss surgery. This membership is a one-stop shop where all your post-op weight loss surgery needs are met in one place.

Pink text-based logo of the T.R.I.B.E. Membership program with images of a computer screen and handouts that are available within the program. Text below the image reads "The T.R.I.B.E.™ Membership is a self-paced, step-by-step membership for babes pre- and post-weight loss surgery. This membership is a one-stop shop where all your post-op weight loss surgery needs are met in one place."

Scan the QR code below or head to
https://thesleeveddietitian.com/the-tribe-membership to join!

And as a very special thank you to you for reading this book and being here on this journey with me I would love for you to use CODE: ITSNOTEASY for 15% off your first subscription.

QR code that can be scanned with a phone or other camera-enabled device. To access the sam materials, visit www.thesleevedditition.com/the-tribe-membership with a discount code ITSNO TEASY for 15% off your first subscription.

The Sleeved Dietitian® acknowledges that the acronym for our community T.R.I.B.E.® is the same as a word used to describe many different indigenous communities. We honor the similarity through our commitment to DEIB (diversity, equity, inclusion, and belonging) and are always open to conversations around identity and inclusion. To lear more about the creation of the T.R.I.B.E.® and how our community came to be, please visit our website www.thesleeveddietitian.com.

Printed in the USA
CPSIA information can be obtained
at www.ICGtesting.com
LVHW020820070923
757252LV00012B/293/J

9 798988 600305